The Definitive Guide to Disc Golf

Justin Menickelli, PhD
and Ryan "Slim" Pickens, MA

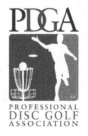

PROFESSIONAL
DISC GOLF
ASSOCIATION

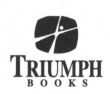

TRIUMPH
BOOKS

This book is available in quantity at special discounts for your group or organization. For further information, contact:

Triumph Books LLC
814 North Franklin Street
Chicago, Illinois 60610
(312) 337-0747
www.triumphbooks.com

Printed in U.S.A.
ISBN: 978-1-62937-204-4
Design by Patricia Frey

This book is officially endorsed by the Professional Disc Golf Association.

This book is dedicated to
Kristin, Aidan, Noah, Addison, Kelly, and Ellora Don.

Contents

Part II: The Science of the Game

Part III: The Skills of the Game

Preface

What Makes Disc Golf a Great Lifetime Sport?

For people just starting to play, disc golf may become an outdoor sport they can enjoy for a lifetime. Mark Twain ostensibly referred to traditional golf (played with a little white ball) as "a good walk spoiled." We like to think of disc golf as "a good walk defined," because it can be appreciated by people of all ages and ability. Men and women, boys and girls can exercise and socialize during a round of disc golf. Avid disc golfers often find playing a challenging test of both physical skill and mental determination. Much like playing traditional golf, the physical and mental challenges great disc golf courses offer are not only enjoyable, but positively addictive.

There are many qualities that make disc golf appealing. For one, playing disc golf is a much less time-consuming alternative to traditional golf. It is also a greener sport than most, as it does not require devastation of natural resources or use of pesticides. Disc golf is an inexpensive lifetime sport; compared to other sports, the start-up cost is minimal. After all, you can play with a single disc that costs about $10. Most of the 4,000 or so disc golf courses in the US are open to the public and free to play. There is a lot of debate over whether or not pay-to-play is the future of the sport, but for now, it is hard to beat free.

In addition to all those positives, playing disc golf is a healthy form of exercise. We know this, in part, because we conducted a nationwide study to discover if playing disc golf was a way for people to walk 10,000 steps a day, the amount recommended to maintain a healthy cardiovascular system. We discovered that each time people venture outside to play disc golf, they take an average of just more than 6,000 steps. Combine a few hours of disc golf with the 5,000 or so steps the average person already walks each day, and we can reap the benefits of sustained, low- to moderate-intensity aerobic exercise. A working heart is a happy one.

Why This Book?

Much more than just a basic "how-to," we think readers will find this book a thoughtful, fascinating, and thoroughly enjoyable exploration of the nature, science, and skills of disc golf. After reading dozens of books about archery, backpacking, badminton, boating, bowling, cycling, fishing, golf, running, skiing, swimming, tennis, and Ultimate, we were inspired to write a comprehensive book about disc golf that would be enjoyed by all players, from absolute beginners to aspiring professionals. There is a lot of information (some of it incorrect or confusing) about disc golf on the Internet. We made it our mission to present technical and accurate content written in a casual voice. Our goal was to write engaging prose that begs to be read cover to cover, and to provide readers with a helpful resource that warrants keeping a copy close by to reference.

We had the privilege of speaking with hundreds of amateur and professional players, course designers, teachers, tournament directors, equipment manufacturers, and living legends of the game. It was a real learning experience for us, and we tried to share this unique perspective throughout the book. Readers may sense a regional bias in some chapters. Although we have played courses and tournaments across the US and the world, we are lucky to live in western North Carolina, a great place to play disc golf, and we could not help but let this shine through in this book.

Acknowledgments

From Justin: I would like to thank all the members of the Catamount Disc Golf Club in Cullowhee, North Carolina, especially Eric Romaniczyn, Clark Lipkin, Andrew Judson, Mike Faust, and Drew Cook. Thanks to all the great people in the WNC Disc Golf Association, including Chris Tuten, Nate Kellar, and James Nichols. Thanks to the EDGE crew: Jay Reading, Des Reading, David Shope, and Jon Lyksett. Thanks to David Claxton, Chris Cooper, Dan Grube, and my students from Western Carolina University. Last, thanks to my family (especially Kristin) and friends who helped make this project a success.

From Ryan: I would like to thank the talented crew of players who helped create Seven Oaks, Two Rivers, and Cedar Hill disc golf courses in Nashville, Tennessee—especially Tuna, Johnny, Ben, Ken, Bob V., Brett, and Farm Fresh. Thanks to all the members of both the WNC Disc Golf Association and the Lakefront Disc Golf Association who, through countless hours of volunteer work, have truly made the western North Carolina / eastern Tennessee region one of the best places to play disc golf in the world.

Thanks to the countless players over the years whom I have had the pleasure to know and who have helped me understand a thing or two. Thanks also to the legend, Ted Williams, who reminded me that God is always on the fairway, and to my longtime doubles partner, Eric Marx, who frequently demonstrates that age does not dictate your score and that whining while winning is pretty annoying. I love you, Marx. Thanks to my late friend Jerry Harmon, who showed me the elevator putt worked and that pouring tee pads is not for the weak. Thank you, Jerry. Thanks also to all my fierce competitors who execute shots that are truly special to witness; you have taught me that losing can still be fun. Last, thanks to my parents, wife, and best friends, who have always believed in me and provided support, which has helped make both this book and my life success.

From Justin and Ryan: We would both like to thank the folks at the Professional Disc Golf Association, especially Dan "Stork" Roddick, for their tremendous support and endorsement of this book. Thanks also to the photographers, the manufacturers that provided photographs, and to the photographic models. Last, thanks to hundreds of players, fans, course designers, tournament directors, and legends of the game for giving their time to be interviewed.

Part I

The Nature of the Game

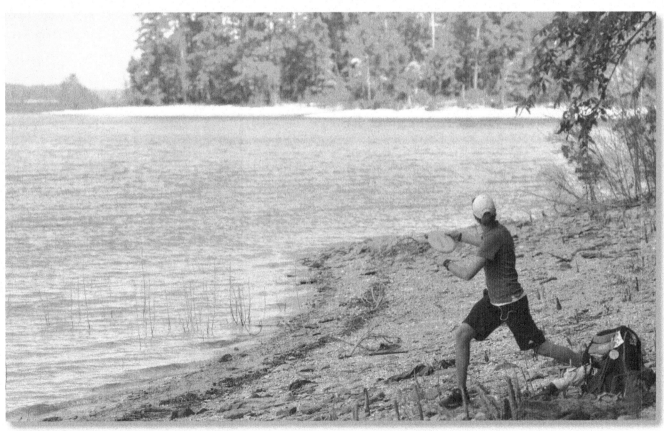

Sara Nicholson's approach throw on hole 14 of the Steady Ed Headrick Memorial Course at the International Disc Golf Center in Appling, Georgia. *Photo courtesy of PDGA Media*

Chapter 1

Getting Started

Technically, the proper name of the sport is disc golf, although some people call it Frisbee golf or, oftentimes in jest, frolf. The primary goal of disc golf is a simple one: to complete the course in the fewest number of throws possible. The basic rules, strategies, and lingo in disc golf are similar to those of traditional golf. In fact, we have lengthy conversations with colleagues who are avid traditional golfers, and if you were to eavesdrop on our dialogue, you would have no idea we were talking about different sports. Terms like *course, hole, par, bogey, birdie, putt, drive, **fairway**,* and *green* are common to both.

Players may choose to compete against other people, but in the end they really just total their number of throws and compare it to the number of throws other players needed to complete the same course. There is a great deal of strategy involved, but very little of it has to do with what fellow competitors are doing, except during the last few **holes** of tournament play. Some engaging competition can bring out your best possible game, but strategizing your way around a disc golf course is primarily about personal shot selection, which we will talk about in upcoming chapters.

Disc golf is considered a lifetime sport because people often play well into their seventies. It is an **individual lifetime sport** and differs from **dual lifetime sports** in the basic cognitive strategies used during play. Dual lifetime sports are those you perform with just one other person (the person against whom you are competing) or with a partner against another pair. Dual lifetime sports include racket sports (e.g., tennis, badminton, squash, and racquetball) and combat sports (e.g., judo and fencing). When playing dual lifetime sports, your opponent may dictate your skill execution, especially if you are getting beaten badly. While playing disc golf, your next shot is almost never dictated by anyone other than yourself, as your thoughts and behaviors are all that really matter.

In disc golf, spectacular shots are often rewarded. Sure, you may get a bad or good skip off a tree, but consistently good throws often translate to better scores, particularly on well-designed courses. When playing dual sports, great execution is rewarded, but because you are facing an opponent capable of defensive tactics, it is just not the same. When playing disc golf, great shots can be stored in your memory for years and retrieved when you need a good image to get you excited about playing. As our friend Boomer once said, "You hold on to the great ones." Someone once told us that both traditional and disc golfers play against the same opponent every time: themselves. We like to think we play against **par** every time, but it is pretty much you against the course.

Choosing the Best Equipment, Footwear, and Clothing

We will discuss **disc** selection as it relates to the physics of disc flight later, but first we want to mention *where* to buy discs and the basic equipment needed to play. When feasible, we encourage people to buy from local, mom-and-pop disc golf shops, but there are several reputable online retailers. Some brick-and-mortar disc golf specialty shops even let you test-throw before you purchase. Specialty disc golf stores are typically great places to shop because of their varied selection and knowledgeable sales staff. For the price of the average traditional golf driver, you can purchase around 20 disc golf drivers. Because discs are relatively inexpensive, typically from $9 to around $18, trying new discs (particularly drivers) is a fun part of the sport. Manufacturers know this and release new drivers every few months that promise greater distance off the tee with less effort.

Let us state what seems obvious to avid players: you are going to want to play with discs designed specifically for disc golf. We remember our friends Andrew and Eric claiming they wanted to start playing disc golf, but that they wanted to keep things simple and play with a single disc designed for throwing and catching. We all laugh about it now, because they each have hundreds of golf discs.

If you are an avid **Ultimate** player, then you are accustomed to throwing discs designed to throw and catch. Golf discs are different, in part because they tend to fly much farther, and most are not easy or safe to catch. There is a bit of a learning curve when transitioning from one type of disc to another, but trust us—it will not take long to learn the basic technique and begin enjoying disc golf. Folks new to disc sports are often intrigued by how throwing different discs the same way results in unique flight patterns.

How many discs do players typically carry during a round? The average is around 20. Some people, like our friend Vinny, play with many different sets of discs. Sometimes he plays with discs from a single manufacturer, and he even has sets organized solely by color. Most players have a primary set of discs and may swap out a few depending on the type of course they are playing. In addition to different flight patterns, some discs take on sentimental value, especially those that seem to find their **target** in glorious ways.

Of course, to carry all of those discs, every player needs a good bag. We strongly recommend a bag that is specifically designed to carry golf discs and is at least one size larger than you think you will need. Why not simply use an old backpack? You could do that, but disc golf–specific ones just seem to work better, largely because you can easily see and retrieve a disc for a particular shot.

Disc golf bags come in a wide variety of sizes and colors, and prices range from around $30 to more than $300. Some bags resemble backpacks and some look more like big nylon boxes. Either way, we strongly recommend getting one with two back straps. You will end up carrying other items in your bag, and that is why we think larger is better. Upon completely emptying one of our bags, we unearthed 23 discs, 2 water bottles, 2 towels for disc drying, a lightweight jacket, a chalk bag (for better **grip** when it gets hot outside), an old pair of sunglasses, insect repellent, sunscreen, 2 mini discs (for marking our **lie**), a permanent black marker, a small bag of sunflower seeds, a half-eaten granola bar, a pair of nail clippers, a very old deck of playing cards, two bag tags, a rule book, five used scorecards from three different courses, three small pencils, and $1.78 in change.

If you dress for a sturdy walk outdoors, then you are more than 90 percent ready to play disc golf. It is essential to wear loose-fitting, comfortable shirts and shorts or pants that allow for full range of motion when walking and throwing. In the summer, many players choose to wear a visor or hat to shade the sun from their eyes, and in the winter, they opt for a warm hat. Most players prefer to wear some type of synthetic wicking fiber shirt when it is hot outside. Some players wear knee-high socks to guard against poison ivy. When we see people playing disc golf in jeans, we shake our heads and wonder how they can possibly be comfortable. We suspect really baggy jeans might be fine when it is cold outside. When the weather turns cold or rainy, it's a good idea to pack a lightweight, waterproof jacket or vest. A warm, synthetic base layer and a windproof fleece vest are great for winter play. These are some popular choices among disc golfers, but during casual play, you can basically wear whatever you want.

Footwear is a critical part of playing many sports, and this is true of disc golf. A lot of players choose to wear hiking shoes. Waterproof versions are, of course, best to wear when precipitation is an issue, but some of the heavier versions can feel a bit clunky. One issue unique to disc golf is that the very best shoes to wear for driving from **tee pads** are not the best for trouncing through the woods or walking on slick grass. Tee pads are used to designate the area from which players must drive and are often made of concrete. Some players prefer to wear soccer-type cleats when playing on natural tee pads. Cleats on concrete tee pads can be slippery and dangerous. Some players, like our friend James, choose to wear high-top hiking boots, and since James is a big, strong guy who always throws from a standstill, we can reason why. Court shoes designed for tennis or basketball work well on concrete tee pads but not as well on the trail. Sandals with open toes are risky because, in addition to the lack of lateral support, many players drag their non-plant foot and thus risk a toe injury when wearing them. Some companies do sell disc golf–specific footwear, but to us they look and perform similar to most lightweight hiking shoes. Sturdy, sweat-wicking synthetic socks are a must. Some players prefer to wear two thin pairs with some cornstarch powder in between layers. Again, the choice is ultimately up to you.

This last piece of equipment falls in the *nonessential* category, but if you really want to improve your game, owning one is critical. Every aspiring disc golfer should acquire a portable target (also called a **basket**) to practice **putting** and **upshots**. There is no greater bang for the buck in the disc golf world, perhaps even the entire sporting world. A very nice target designed for temporary holes and practice costs just less than $200. If you have a 40'x40' parcel of land and a disc golf target, then you have a worthy putting **green**. One of our oldest friends, an avid traditional golfer, has a modest golf putting green in his backyard. It took 100 or more hours of construction, more than a ton of materials (rock, sand, sod, drainage pipes, and wood for the border), and about $8,000 to devise this roughly 25'x25' putting green. The special mower he uses to cut the grass cost him another $2,000, and he is constantly running his kids off the green.

Types of Golf and Tournament Play

Rounds of disc golf are inherently different. Some days you might simply want to play a casual round with friends. Many players use casual rounds to practice different throwing techniques or focus on aspects of their game that need improvement. During tournament play, players take their games more seriously in an effort to score well. Understanding that there are inherently different types of disc golf may enhance your own golf experience and your respect for other golfers. Rick Kapalko may have described this experience best when he cleverly defined four types of disc golf: soul, practice, fun, and tournament golf.

Kapalko's description of soul golf sounds like what we refer to as disc golf Zen. There are indeed days, rounds, holes, throws, and moments in time that seem to transcend disc golf reality. For example, during a mystical round of **glow golf** (a game played at night with illuminated plastic discs or ones with glowing sticks affixed to their tops), our friend Drew once reached disc golf Zen. It was a chilly night, there was a full moon in the sky, and a frosty mist seemed to permeate the evening air. The weather conditions did not warrant low scores, but Drew holed out every throw inside 80 feet. He seemed to be in a soulful state of deep **flow** or Zen. All he could do was chuckle in bewilderment, and we all laughed as well. By definition, deeply soulful rounds of disc golf are rare and difficult to define. They are often played with friends, but playing by yourself can also elicit such experiences.

Practice golf is just that: good practice. You might throw a new disc, try new throwing styles, or focus on improving your technique. Some people like to go to an open field to practice throws, and that is a great idea. During practice rounds, a person might throw two putts from every lie and may not keep score. We suppose that having fun during practice golf is not essential, but if you are not a disc golf professional, you have the luxury of quitting a practice round when you are simply not having fun. Many players never practice, but as you will learn in upcoming chapters, practice golf is the best way to develop consistency in your game.

Fun golf includes games like **Wolf** (more about Wolf in appendix A) or Ript Revenge, an amusing disc golf / card game where you may have to throw with your non-dominant arm or from another player's lie. During fun golf, you might heckle other players, and your score probably matters very little. We think both **target** and **safari golf** are part of fun golf. In target golf, targets such as trees or signs are used in lieu of formal targets. If you hit the intended tree, then you have holed out. Mapping out a course though a college campus, urban area, neighborhood, or some woods can be really adventurous, provided safety is paramount. A lot of people began playing target golf before a formal course was built in their area. Safari golf can be played on either a target or permanent course. During safari golf, impromptu holes are often chosen by the group. For example, you might **drive** from the tee pad on hole 3 to the target on hole 6. Playing safari golf can be quite adventurous, much like you are on a safari.

During tournament golf, all the official rules of disc golf apply. There are no **mulligans**, no gimme putts, and you must keep score meticulously. We have no data to support the notion that playing in tournaments leads to consistently better scores, but nearly everyone we spoke with claimed that it makes you a better disc golfer. Some people think weekly club-sponsored events are under the umbrella of tournament play, and they are probably right. Clubs typically host weekly singles and doubles events, and in larger clubs they can be as competitive as sanctioned tournaments. There are a few sanctioned doubles tournaments in which you often bring your own partner. More about tournament play later.

The types of disc golf are not mutually exclusive. For example, tournament golf can be soulful, fun, and just plain good practice. For people new to playing disc golf, all rounds might be casual and fun. If you are just starting to play disc golf, the thought of playing in a tournament may be overwhelming, but rest assured it can be exciting and challenging in a competitive but nonthreatening way.

Tournament Tiers and Player Divisions

Playing in tournaments is a great way to improve your game, meet up with old friends, and make new friends who share your passion

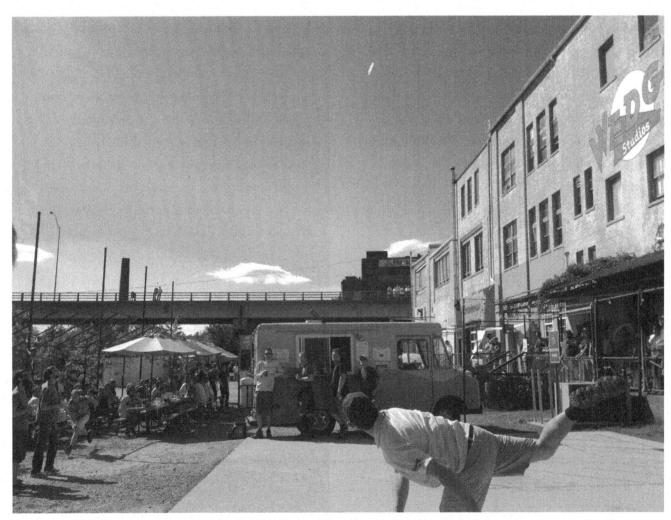

Henry Childress at the Wedge Brewing Company in Asheville, North Carolina, throwing over a food truck to a temporary target on the overpass. *Photo by Jenny Ung Urroz*

for disc golf. Tournament tiers and player divisions, as established by the Professional Disc Golf Association (PDGA), are pretty easy to comprehend, even for someone who knows little about the organizational structure. Of course, you can find all the details at www.pdga.com.

Local tournaments tend to have a mellow vibe, and the competition, particularly in the recreational divisions, may be less intense than larger events. They are a great place for large numbers of local club players to represent the club. One of our favorite tournaments is the Mountain Disc Golf Experience, which takes place annually in Asheville, North Carolina. It is a great tournament, at least in part, because of its unique events. On Saturday, the top amateur players play nine holes around the site of the popular Mountain Sports Festival. On Sunday, the best professionals play a **skins** event through crowded downtown streets. Players often tee off from the tops of buildings and throw over hundreds of spectators to precarious target placements.

Membership in the PDGA

To play in most tournaments, you do not have to be a member of the PDGA. If you choose to play more than a handful of tournaments a year, it makes

financial sense to join, because you very often pay a discounted entry fee for being a member. In addition to discounts, members are assigned an official player number and earn a player rating. Basically, your **PDGA Player Rating** is a number that represents how close your average round scores are compared to the course ratings, called the **Scratch Scoring Average**, of the courses you have played during officially sanctioned tournaments. Players rated exactly 1,000 are considered scratch players. Scratch players are almost always highly skilled professionals.

A lot of people prefer to play casual rounds and local doubles events instead of sanctioned tournaments. Many of the million or so avid players cannot name more than one touring professional and many are not members of the PDGA. For us, being part of an organization means more than the bottom line, and being active members makes us feel like we are part of something bigger. If you are serious about improving your game or want to contribute to making the sport better, we strongly encourage you to become an active member of a local club and the PDGA.

Chapter 2

The History, Present, and Possible Future of Disc Golf

On August 12, 2002, "Steady" Ed Headrick, the designer of the modern Frisbee and "the father of disc golf," died at his home in La Selva Beach, California, at the age of 78. As stipulated in his will, Headrick's remains were cremated and his ashes were molded into a limited number of Frisbees, ensuring he would be flying through the air for years to come. Most of the discs were given to his friends and family and the remainder were sold, with all proceeds going to a nonprofit fund to build a Steady Ed Memorial Disc Golf Museum. Headrick's dream of better flying discs continues to influence many others who help make throwing Frisbee discs more than simply a playful distraction.

The Evolution of the Frisbee

The origins of flying objects that resemble modern discs can be traced to the early 1870s and Bridgeport, Connecticut. Locals and students at nearby Yale University took to tossing empty tin pie plates from the Frisbie Pie Company owned by William Russell Frisbie. The pie plates, dubbed frisbies, were readily available, sturdy, easy to catch, and flew quite well for an object designed to hold pie. Over the next five decades, throwing and catching pie plates for fun spread across the US, and following the Depression, they were a lot cheaper than baseballs. Recycling efforts during the World War II era may have put a damper on "frisbieing," but the development of flexible, moldable plastics soon changed the world forever.

One of the companies to benefit from technological advances in plastics was Wham-O Mfg. Co. in San Gabriel, California. In 1956 Walter Fredrick Morrison approached Wham-O about the plastic "flying saucer" he and others had first created a decade before. Morrison offered to sell his design to Wham-O executives for $25,000, but they balked at the chance and instead offered him future royalties on all flying discs sold by the company. In 1957 Wham-O sold its first disc designed by Morrison and dubbed it the **Pluto Platter** in an effort to profit from America's obsession with space and flying saucers. The Pluto Platter was soft, easy to catch, and had a predictable flight, providing that the thrower did not try to toss it very far and there was little wind. Because of Morrison's contract with Wham-O, he eventually profited more than a million dollars from the future sales of flying discs. The next decade would prove to be a landmark one in the development of the Frisbee.

By the mid 1960s, the Hula-Hoop fad was fading a bit and Wham-O needed a new toy gadget. Ed Headrick was a resourceful, hardworking World War II veteran in the right place at the right time. Headrick even convinced Wham-O he would work for free until he was worthy of compensation. He did not take long to prove his worth, and in 1964 he created the Pro Model Frisbee by completely redesigning the Pluto Platter. Headrick used stiffer plastics and incorporated concentric, grooved lines into the top of Frisbees in an effort to increase stability (resistance to **flipping**) during flight.

The newly designed Frisbees, with the "lines of Headrick," were more aerodynamic and flew much farther and with greater accuracy than the Pluto Platter. In essence, they felt more like a piece of sporting equipment and less like a toy. Flying Frisbees quickly became popular sights on beaches and in parks. Flashy, acrobatic throwing and catching, or "freestyling," became the hip recreational activity, particularly in the western states. A game called **guts**, in which players throw a disc as fast as possible (so as not to be caught) at an opposing five-person team, grew to be the most popular competition played with a Frisbee. To spread the joy of flying Frisbees across the US, it would take more than a new design, though.

Headrick was outgoing, determined, and exceptionally good at his job. To market this new piece of sporting equipment, Headrick formed the International Frisbee Association (IFA) in 1967, an organization that claimed as many as 112,000 members by 1972 (most from California). Ostensibly a Wham-O marketing/promotional tool, the initial mission of the IFA was to promote the

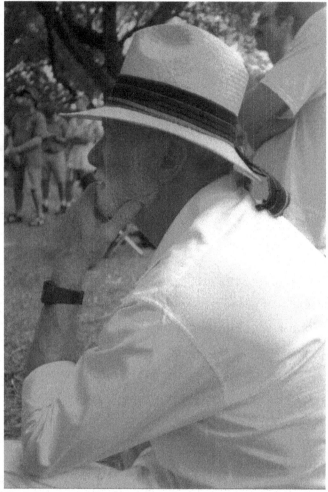

The father of disc golf, "Steady" Ed Headrick. *Photo courtesy of the Disc Golf Association*

sport of guts and ultimately sell more Frisbees. The IFA circulated a newsletter in 1968 that reached many folks in the western US. Although the circulation was not far-reaching, the importance of this first newsletter to eventually promote all sports played with a Frisbee should not be overlooked.

Disc Golf Takes Flight

Exactly who invented the game of disc golf is unclear. There were certainly many people who began playing unique versions of the modern game prior to the 1960s. A game called Sky Golf that used croquet wicket–like targets was available from Copar Plastics company in 1960. In 1961 Kevin Donnelly set up a six-hole Frisbee golf course at the 38th Street Park in Newport Beach, California, using trees and light poles as targets. Attendance at the park grew rapidly because of Donnelly's target course, and by the next year, two other city parks had courses and Donnelly organized monthly competitions. In 1965 Donnelly asked Wham-O executives to sponsor the first Frisbee disc golf tournament at Mariners Park in Newport Beach. They agreed and sent him 100 of Headrick's Pro Model Frisbees along with 24 Hula-Hoops to use as targets. In preparation for the tournament, Donnelly developed the first set of formal Frisbee golf rules and tournament director responsibilities. In 1966 Donnelly began teaching recreational activities at Fresno State College. While lecturing about Frisbee golf, an astute senior in his class raised his hand and said, "I have played that game too." That student was a man named George Sappenfield, who coincidentally had worked part-time for Wham-O from 1964 to 1965.

In 1968 Sappenfield graduated from Fresno State and became the recreation supervisor at a park in Thousand Oaks, California. The next year, he planned an event that closely resembled modern disc golf, and like his professor, he contacted Wham-O to supply Frisbees and Hula-Hoops. But Sappenfield went one step further. Using a connection from his brief employ at Wham-O, he convinced Headrick to include Frisbee golf as part of the popular Frisbee skills competition that Wham-O was planning to stage at Brookside Park in Pasadena, California. The competition featured events such as freestyle and throwing for maximum distance. They agreed. About 40 people played the nine-hole round of Frisbee golf, many of whom did not play the round competitively but simply gave it a try. The winner of the Frisbee golf event was UC Berkeley student Jay Shelton. Shelton and others brought the game back to Berkeley, where it became a popular activity on a campus already known for flying discs. Sappenfield eventually worked full-time for Wham-O from 1979 to 1985, continuing to greatly influence the growth of the sport.

In 1970 a group of people from Rochester, New York, who were not familiar with the IFA or the Frisbee golf happenings on the West Coast began playing an organized, competitive version of disc golf. They had their own newsletter, called the *Rochester Frisbee Club Newsletter*. One of the disc golf fanatics from Rochester was also an avid ball golfer named Jim Palmeri. During the early days, Palmeri and others used square wooden baskets that had once held wine bottles as targets on the ground. The Continental Promotions Inc. (CPI) All-Star, and not Headrick's popular Pro Model Frisbee, was their disc of choice. In 1971 they began promoting a citywide championship, and by 1974, after reading an IFA newsletter, they decided to make their citywide event a national tournament.

They called the tournament the American Flying Disc Open because the Rochester contingent was informed via the IFA newsletter that Wham-O had trademarked the term *Frisbee*. They announced they would award a 1974 Datsun B210 automobile to the winner of a combined event: disc golf and double-disc court (a game that resembled both volleyball and tennis but was played with two discs). Folks from all over the country came to play in this first national tournament. The winner was Dan "Stork" Roddick, whom Headrick subsequently hired to work for Wham-O and promote the sport. Roddick was a Rutgers University graduate student and freestyling phenom. He was very tall and athletic, and in short-shorts and tube socks (en vogue at the time), he strongly resembled his nickname.

Later that year the 1974 World Frisbee Championships did not include a disc golf competition because Wham-O was not yet vested in promoting the sport. However, Roddick, Sappenfield, Palmeri, and others urged Headrick to include disc golf as part of the forthcoming 1975 World Frisbee Championships at the Rose Bowl in Pasadena, California. The first temporary course was put in place for this event at nearby Oak Grove Park in Pasadena, California.

Better Targets and Big Promotions

Steady Ed had a busy and prosperous year in 1975. Three key developments, all credited to him, spurred the growth of the sport. He formed the Professional Disc Golf Association as a means for promoting the sport of disc golf by sanctioning professional tournaments, and he designed what most people believe to be the first formal disc golf course, at Oak Grove Park in Pasadena, California.

Perhaps the most notable development was Headrick's target called a **Pole-hole,** which helped to standardize the game and became the

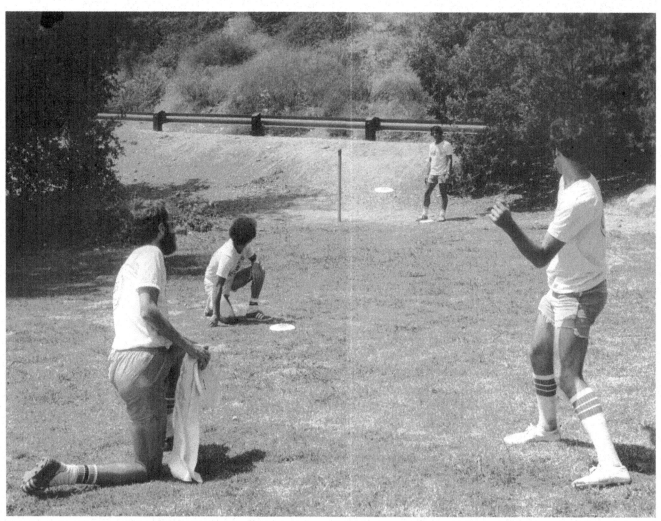

Hole 10 at the 1975 World Frisbee Championships at Oak Grove. Pictured from left to right are Dan Roddick, Jim Palmeri, Jimmy Scala, and Irv Kalb. *Photo courtesy of the IFA*

equivalent of the hole/pin/flag combination used in traditional golf. Players in the western states were predominantly using four-foot vertical poles as targets. The issue with using poles was that it was difficult to tell if a player holed out (hit the pole). Players had to see or hear a disc hit the pole, and from 50 feet away that was very difficult to do. Players in the eastern states were predominantly using ground baskets. It was easy to tell if the disc came to rest in the basket but it allowed players to roll or throw a disc vertically in an effort to "spike" or "drop" the disc in the basket (Roddick's specialty). He despised this vertical putting style but liked the idea of definitive hole-outs, so he wisely combined the two popular targets into one. Headrick created the Pole-hole in secret in an effort to keep others from duplicating his design.

Headrick hired Roddick to be the director of the IFA. One of Roddick's first tasks was to meet with Tom Monroe from Huntsville, Alabama, and ask him to be an IFA regional director. Monroe was issued a Wham-O company car (a customized Dodge van) in which to travel all over the country and spread the joy of Frisbee sports. Monroe assembled a demonstration team, called Frisbee South, which traveled the US visiting public schools and college campuses. They performed freestyle shows and guts demonstrations at Major League Baseball games, NASCAR races, and NBA basketball games.

In an effort to promote the burgeoning sport of disc golf, Roddick later began to develop, promote, and manage the 1975 North American Series as qualifying tournaments for the World Frisbee Championships. The tour was essentially a traveling circus of agile hippies driving Volkswagen Microbuses to festivals in places like Seattle, San Diego, St. Louis, Boston, and Sarasota, Florida. The events introduced disc golf to thousands of traditional Frisbee throwers and helped create a sustainable market for Headrick to sell Frisbees and Pole-holes across the country.

Headrick was a complex, often obsessive man and a talented inventor. He added chains and a basket to his Pole-hole (some folks in Rochester were still using baskets). His new target, called the Chain Pole-hole, eliminated the difficulty of determining if a Pole-hole had been hit because the disc could come to rest in the basket, indicating the player had successfully holed out. The chains also had a dampening or "catching" effect when a disc hit them. Headrick was not alone in his efforts to create Frisbee golf targets. In St. Paul, Minnesota, Ken Krengel and Jim Challas designed a space-age-looking target dubbed a Saucer Golf target in 1977, but Headrick's Chain Pole-hole set the new standard—in large part because it was simply a better target.

Finally convinced that disc golf had the potential to be a viable and profitable sport, Headrick boldly resigned from his position at Wham-O and started his own company, the Disc Golf Association (DGA), in 1976. Headrick set up on-course shops run by handpicked professionals to sell his newly designed discs and Chain Pole-holes. One such professional was a skillful player named Snapper Pierson, who started operating a pro shop at the Morley Field course in San Diego, California, in 1977. The course is one of the most frequently played disc golf courses today and is still operated by Pierson. While the sport of disc golf took root, the development of better flying discs continued at a rapid rate.

Better Flying Discs

By 1978 there was a growing market for flying discs to be used in a variety of games. An avid freestyle player named Jim Kenner formed a London, Ontario–based company with the idea of producing both golf discs (designed to be thrown but not caught) and freestyle discs (designed to be thrown and caught). In fact, Kenner is credited with developing the first discs designed specifically for freestyle play. His company, Discraft, later moved to Wixom, Michigan, in 1981 and introduced a milestone disc. The Ultra-Star, a great throw-and-catch disc, was a favorite among the growing number of people playing a fast-paced game that resembled soccer called Ultimate. A decade later, it became the official disc of the Ultimate Players Association (now called USA Ultimate). In the late 1970s Kenner was not the only person trying to design and sell better flying discs for the fledgling sport of disc golf.

Jan "Whizbo" Sobel, a long-haired, free-spirited entrepreneur from Hollywood, California, designed a very heavy disc for its time (200 grams and heavier) that he began selling out of the trunk of his car around 1981 in an effort to provide flying discs to the growing disc golf market. Sobel's disc, called the Puppy, was a huge hit among disc golfers and would later prove to be a landmark design. In the days before weight limits, the heavy Puppy was considered by many to be the best all-around golf disc. Sobel followed his success with a disc called the Super Puppy. Sobel's sophomore effort was even more popular, likely because there were more potential players to throw it. He later released another popular disc called the Floater that he marketed to surf shops on the West Coast like a persistent door-to-door salesman. Sobel certainly left his mark on the sport, as his 21-centimeter disc size is still one of the most popular sizes of discs today.

Ted Smethers, from Little Rock, Arkansas, developed the first professional tour, which began in the summer of 1982; that same year, the first PDGA Disc Golf World Championships was held in Los Angeles, California. In early 1983 Headrick open-sourced his trademarked term *disc golf*, allegedly first coined by Roddick. After a new association called the US Disc Players Golf Association threatened the PDGA stranglehold, Headrick reluctantly relinquished control of the PDGA to the players. A relatively unknown regional pro, Smethers became the first commissioner of the PDGA in 1983. Later, at the 1984 Worlds in Rochester, New York, Headrick symbolically handed over the PDGA to Smethers with a handshake and a can of locally brewed Genesee Cream Ale. With the newly organized PDGA governing the growing sport, the hunger for better-designed discs—and tasty hamburgers—would change the sport forever.

Harold Duvall was in line to get a hamburger with his brother Charlie during a Frisbee skills tournament when Dave Dunipace overheard them talking about finding someone to play in a pickup game of basketball. As it turned out, Dunipace was looking for some disc golf playing partners as well. At the time, guts and double-disc court still had a significantly more prominent place in Frisbee skills tournaments than disc golf. Harold Duvall was fresh off playing in his first disc golf tournament, the 1982 World Championships, which he won. The Duvall brothers and Dunipace (who had placed second in the 1982 Worlds) dreamed of a better golf disc. Together they convinced Tim Selinske to leave his marketing position at Wham-O to take aim at their dream, and Innova Champion Discs was born in 1983. Selinske (Ske to his friends) was perhaps best known for his big, mustache-boosted smile. Selinske did more than answer the phones at the fledgling company's office, he became their public relations guru. The much-beloved Selinske later died of cancer, in 2009.

The early to mid 1980s brought a revolution in disc design. In 1983 Dunipace, a pioneer of golf disc design, created what is considered by most people to be the first true golf disc: the Innova Eagle (later called the Aero). The Eagle was the first disc that a person would not dare try to catch. With a low-profile rim, it flew much farther than any other disc available and could never be mistaken for a Puppy or an Ultra-Star. The Eagle helped disc golf evolve from a simple game to a bona fide sport.

Discraft followed suit when they revealed their first disc made specifically for disc golf, called the Phantom, that same year. In 1984 Innova released the first true disc golf putter, called the Aviar. During the 1980s the number of courses began to grow significantly while Innova's own version of the Pole-hole (with more chains to "catch" an approaching disc), began sprouting up on courses across the US.

During the mid to late 1980s, there was a transition from Frisbee skill tournaments—with competitions such as throwing for distance, maximum time aloft, and freestyling—to disc golf–only tournaments. Better, golf-specific flying discs yielded longer throws and ultimately longer courses. Most of the people playing in the tour events were quasi-local, but there were a few

die-hards who would travel to as many events as they could during the summer months. Players including Sam Ferrans (the 1984 world champion) and Gregg Hosfeld (the 1987 world champion) would drive to each city in an aging Dodge conversion van with the goal of making enough money through prize winnings to put gas in the tank and burritos in their bellies. During the early days of the Frisbee tour, everyone who played was a professional, because they could earn money for winning or placing well in tournaments. Often, it was cash that went straight into the faded denim pocket of the winner, which was quickly spent on fuel, food, and beer.

In 1987 Innova released their tremendously popular Roc midrange disc. If the Eagle put Innova on the map, then the release of the Roc established control of the growing equipment market.

In 1987 a new annual event also began, and it shaped the sport of disc golf forever. Rick Rothstein, a passionate and intelligent disc golf advocate, wanted to get a group of local disc golfers out for a round in the deep snow in Columbia, Missouri, on the Sunday before the Super Bowl. With the threat of adverse weather looming, he insisted there be "no wimps" and "no excuses." Thirty-four of his playing buddies showed up on that cold January day in 1987 and played in the first Ice Bowl. Rothstein publicized his Ice Bowl event in a magazine he started the following month called *Disc Golf World News*. Word spread quickly, and the number of Ice Bowl events across the US quickly grew. In 1995, the Indianapolis Disc Golf Club used their Ice Bowl to raise money for their local food bank. This act of philanthropy caught on, and the mission of Ice Bowls across the US became to raise money for charitable organizations.

As of 2012, more than $2 million has been raised from these events.

The Professional Tour

Better flying discs were being designed at a rapid rate, and a more structured and prominent tour took hold. The professional tour began without a real grassroots effort to bring disc golf to the masses, a phenomenon that would later come to haunt many who tried to cultivate the sport. Ken Climo from Clearwater, Florida, emerged to dominate the professional tour. Climo had the icy mystique of Tiger Woods and the lanky-smooth mechanics of "Slammin' Sammy" Snead. The player eventually called, simply, Champ by many folks dominated the professional landscape with nine consecutive world championship titles from 1990 to 1998, and he most certainly helped Innova (his corporate sponsor) sell a lot of discs.

In 1999 Harold Duval, Dave Dunipace, and Jonathan Poole created the United States Disc Golf Championship (USDGC) held in Rock Hill, South Carolina. Climo won that inaugural event and later added four more USDGC titles in 2000, 2002, 2004, and 2007. Climo could make his signature disc, a TeeBird, fly in a way no one else could, and he dominated the sport so impressively that the original working title of this book was *Catching Climo.* Of course, there were many players chasing Climo—such as Dave Feldberg, JohnE McCray, Barry Schultz, Eric Marx, Scott Stokely, and the legendary Ron Russell—but in history there can be only one first, and Climo was the first player to rule the professional ranks. Climo now dominates the professional master's division, the rough equivalent of the Legends Tour in traditional golf.

By the mid 1990s, Elaine King from Toronto, Ontario, emerged as the first queen of the sport. A self-described "weekend warrior," she dominated the women's ranks, winning the world championship from 1991 to 1994 and later in 1997. She went on to win the USDGC in 2005 and 2007. King developed a reputation for being unflappable, gracious, and very intelligent. She earned a PhD in analytical chemistry from the University of Toronto in 1990 and served as the PDGA commissioner in 1993. King plays exceptionally well to this day, and won 13 professional tournaments in 2013.

In the early 2000s two players began to take over the professional women's field. Juliana Korver was best known for her graceful form, exceptional shot-making ability, and as a consummate professional. Somewhat reserved but friendly, Korver had a reputation for playing with ice in her veins on Sunday afternoons. Korver won four consecutive PDGA World Championship titles from 1998 to 2001, and again in 2003. Her contemporary, and fellow University of Northern Iowa alumnus, Desiree "Des" Reading, was tall, strong, and uber-athletic. A former collegiate softball pitcher, she was known for her ability to out-drive many of her competitors and later as a clutch putter. Together, Korver and Reading won most of the major tour events, with Reading often playing the proverbial bridesmaid as the world runner-up six times. Reading won her own world titles in 2002, 2005, and 2006 and padded her résumé with three consecutive USDGC titles from 2002 to 2004. Korver rather quietly walked away from the sport in 2009, while Reading continues to collect an RV full of tour hardware to this day.

During the 2000s, there were players who traveled to tournaments all over the US in

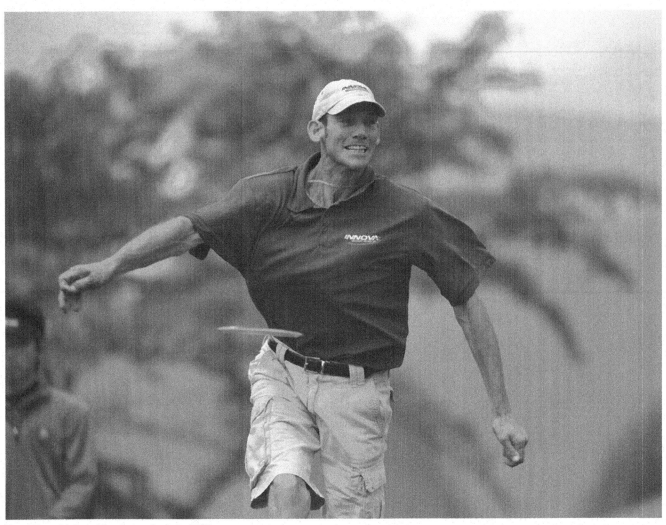

Ken Climo driving at the Japan Open in 2006. *Photo courtesy of Innova Champion Discs*

conversion vans, old Winnebagos, and camper-shelled trucks. They camped close to the tournament site, which brought about increased camaraderie. There was the Winnicrew (Todd Branch, Al Schack, Sue Stephens, Avery Jenkins, David Feldberg, and dog Storm), the Dolphin Crew (Brian Schweberger, Brian McRee, Billy "Nature Boy" Crump, and dog Yukon), Team Reading (Des and Jay Reading), the Flying Eye Crew (Cam Todd, Leslie Herndon, Mike "Worm" Young), Team Spirit (Carrie "Burl" Berlogar, Courtney Peavy, and Val Jenkins), and solo touring players Ron Russell, Kevin McCoy, Brian Mace, Eric McCabe, and Brad Hammock. The tournament winners often bought dinner and drinks for everyone Sunday evening, and there was the mandatory Monday Funday the following day before heading to the next event. Each Monday, the posse of disc golfers would go to the beach, an amusement park, a brewery, or a baseball game. There was no disc golf allowed on Mondays (you could not even mention it), just simple fun and enduring friendship.

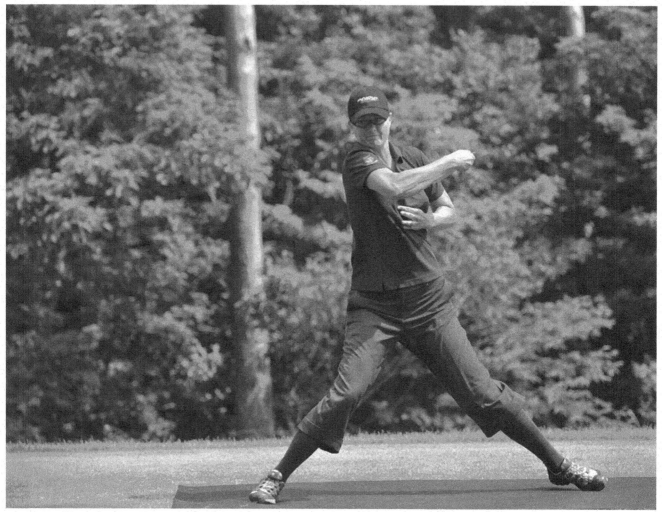

Des Reading's powerful driving form. *Photo courtesy of Innova Champion Discs*

The core Monday Funday crew fizzled out around 2010 as the fresh faces of the sport began touring. The new wave of professionals, with their rocket arms and sponsorships from fledgling companies, preferred to crash on couches rather than camp on-site. Open-house pool parties hosted by people such as Pete Cashen from Kansas City became the new normal, as did connecting with locals via social media instead of face-to-face. Mondays became reserved for traveling to the next event, and practice rounds at the next tournament

stop began a day or two earlier as the tournament fields became deeper and increasingly competitive.

In 2002 Harold Duvall approached Jon Lyksett about an idea to create a nonprofit organization dedicated to providing schools and youth programs a way to teach the skills needed to enjoy playing disc golf. The Educational Disc Golf Experience (EDGE) program was born, and it brought the sport to thousands of young people across the US and the world. The program was financially backed by Innova and staffed only with Innova-sponsored players, prompting some people to refer to EDGE as a brilliant marketing ploy.

In 2003 Discraft developed its own unique promotional strategy by adopting an event that was started by a local club in Ann Arbor, Michigan. The annual event, called the Ace Race, began as a means of promoting a new prototype disc each year. During the event, players typically play modified, shorter holes and try to get as many aces as they can, using only the new prototype. In 2013, dubbed "the largest event in disc golf history," about 20,000 people played in nearly 400 Ace Race events on the same weekend. With more efforts to grow the sport from the bottom up, disc golf needed a place to call home.

In 2007 the PDGA International Disc Golf Center (IDGC)—which houses the "Steady" Ed Memorial Disc Golf Museum, the Disc Golf Hall of Fame, and the PDGA central offices—opened outside of Augusta, Georgia. In addition to giving the PDGA a home base, many people believe the development of the IDGC helped give disc golf a great deal of credibility. Brian Graham, the director of the PDGA from 2007 to the present, is largely credited with making the IDGC possible. The IDGC property also features three spectacular courses designed by legendary course architects Chuck Kennedy, Tom Monroe, John Houck, Jim Kenner, Ron Russell, and Pad Timmons.

The Current State and Possible Future of the Sport

The growth rate of disc golf is staggering. In 1980 there were 60 permanent disc golf courses in the world. In 2013 there were more than 4,500 courses worldwide. From 2003 to 2012, the number of disc golf courses in the US alone grew by 190 percent. Most courses are still located on public land and free to play. Howerever, many people believe that private, pay-to-play courses are the future of the sport.

In its first 35 years of existence, almost 75 percent of traditional ball golf courses were private. By comparison, less than 10 percent of disc golf courses are private. This phenomenon may have resulted in more disc golf courses being constructed than the market demanded. People have come to expect that disc golf courses are free to play. However, by paying a few dollars to play, a player/consumer might come to expect better course design, landscaping, and amenities. As most athletic directors and park managers know, charging a few dollars for an event or service can help create a perception of value. Also, fees from private, pay-to-play courses could be used to supplement tournament payouts. Free public courses will always have their place. They are great for novice players who just want to check out the sport or for youth who want an additional activity to do in the local park.

Today, roughly 10 million people have played disc golf and about 1 million people claim to play regularly. The sport is growing rapidly as the numbers of players roughly doubles every six years. From 2003 to 2012 the number of PDGA-sanctioned tournament competitors in the US grew an astounding 172 percent from 39,382 to 107,006. There are more than 300 disc golf clubs in the US whose members serve to nurture their local courses and cultivate more than 1,800 events worldwide. In 2015 there were 19 major tournaments on the PDGA tour schedule in 14 different states in the US, and in Australia, Finland, and Sweden.

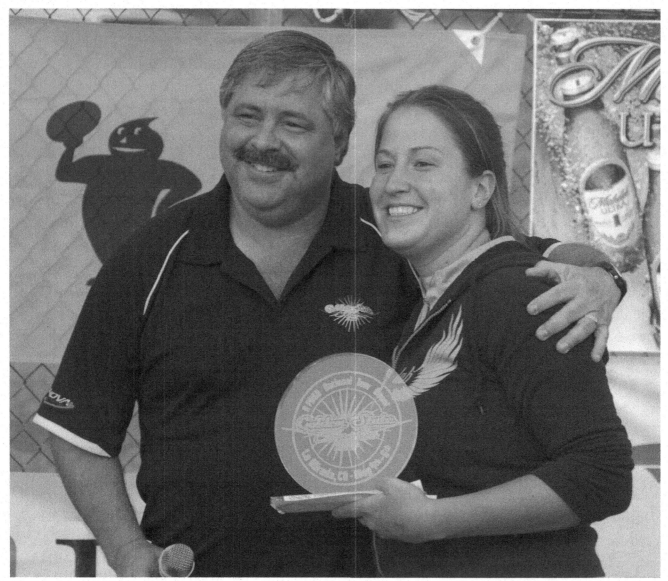

Tim Selinske and Val Jenkins at the 2007 Golden State Classic in La Mirada, California. *Photo courtesy of Innova Champion Discs*

A youth movement comprised primarily of young adults who grew up playing disc golf has taken over the professional ranks. In 2015, a Jordan Spieth–esque young man from Huntington Beach, California, named Paul McBeth dominated the professional field and earned $63,304 in tournament winnings for his efforts while men such as Nikko Locastro, Cale Leiviska, Simon Lizotte, Eric McAbe, Will Shusterick, Paul Ulibarri, Ricki Wysocki, and others gave chase. McBeth established his dominance by winning the PDGA World Championships four times in succession, from 2012 to 2015. His closest contemporary, Will Shusterick from Madison, Tennessee, won the USDGC in 2010, 2012, and 2014.

Two women small in stature but with rocket arms, Minnesotan Catrina Allen and Texan Paige Pierce, have ascended to the top of the women's professional field. In 2015, Pierce won the World Championship, with Allen finishing third. In 2014, Allen claimed the World title (Pierce was second), but Pierce won the U.S. women's title (Allen finished tied for third). Talented and amiable women such as Val Jenkins (the 2007, 2008, and 2009 world champion), Sara Hokom (2012 world champ), Sarah Cunningham (never seen without a Clemson University logo), and others have earned their share of major tournament wins. Interestingly, the top pro women earn about half what their male counterparts earn a year in prize winnings.

Compared to other professional sports, playing disc golf professionally is far from lucrative, and it does not take much to play in a pro tournament field. In fact, anyone can play professionally as long as they write a check and pass a rules examination. There is no qualifying school and no set number of years that person must play in the amateur ranks. Because of this laxity, and with few corporate sponsors to make them accountable for their behavior, more than a few professional players have been known to exhibit discourteous and unprofessional behavior on the course. Many people involved in the sport believe the professional tour is suffering from decades without a grassroots effort to grow the sport from the bottom up. Some professional players contend that reducing the number of tournaments, limiting the pro fields, and increasing the payouts awarded to the winners will result in a top-down growth of the sport.

Many professionals feel they should be compensated more for their talent, which seems pretty reasonable to many fans. However, it will continue to be difficult to make a viable living playing disc golf until tournament highlights consistently make the SportsCenter top 10 list.

If more fans watch tournaments in person, on television, and via the Internet, the PDGA can attract major sponsors, and that, in turn, will produce more revenue. In reality, most people walking the street are amazed anyone can make money by simply playing disc golf.

Competition among equipment manufacturers and the quest for better flying discs continues to affect disc design, but with rigid PDGA technical standards in place, many of the design changes center around developing new blends of plastic as opposed to changes in form. Drivers are often made from very firm plastic and have relatively sharp rim profiles. The general population is under the impression that disc golfers are throwing discs that more closely resemble the throw-and-catch variety, and other stakeholders perpetuate that illusion. The reality is that when someone is struck with a driver disc, serious injury can result. Some people believe the maximum weight of a legal disc for play (200 grams) should be reduced to 159.9 grams (as it is in Japan). All in all, disc golf's safety record over the years has been remarkably good; however, the significant increase in the number of courses could increase the potential for risk. Course designer programs, educational outreach, and disc golf–only facilities will all play a role in the future of the sport, but personal responsibility is paramount.

Disc golf has emerged as a popular global sport. The largest recent growth has been in Scandinavia, with Finland leading the way with more than 300 courses and 700 active PDGA members. During the 2015 European Open in Nokia, an astonishing 26 percent of all TV viewers in Finland tuned in to the live TV broadcast on Sunday afternoon. The PDGA international program—which began in 2004 thanks to the labors of Brian Hoeniger,

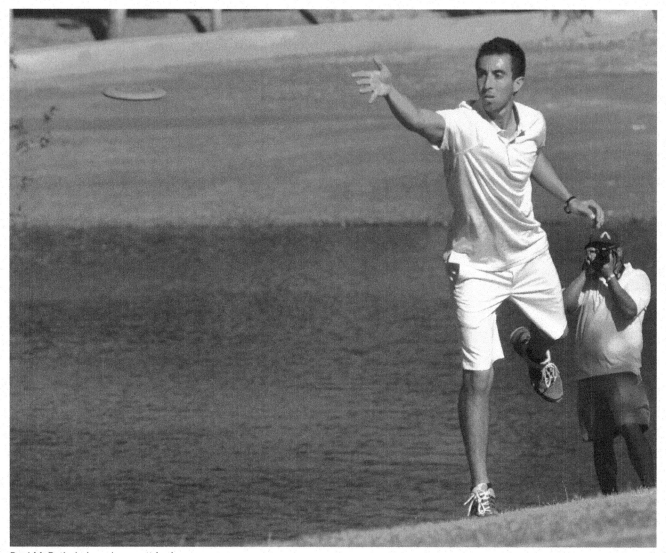

Paul McBeth drains a long putt for fans. *Photo courtesy of PDGA Media*

Dave Nesbitt, and others—was charged with coordinating efforts between the PDGA and national associations throughout the world. There is a thriving European tour, with more than 200 events in places like Belgium, the Czech Republic, Finland, France, Germany, Hungary, Lithuania, the Netherlands, Norway, Spain, Sweden, Switzerland, and the United Kingdom. Open spaces (and thus disc golf courses) are scarce in Japan, but the Japan Open (which began in 1985) is back on the PDGA

Tour schedule after the 2012 cancellation due to the tragic aftermath of the 2011 tsunami.

In 2014 the PDGA rejoined the World Flying Disc Federation (WFDF), regaining its status as a charter member of the WFDF going back to its formation in 1985. Recognized by the International Olympic Committee, the WFDF promotes all flying-disc sports and is composed of national organizations (such as USA Ultimate) and not individual members. A Global Disc Golf

Committee composed of representatives from both the PDGA and the WFDF was formed in an effort to further promote disc golf all over the world. In stark contrast to the governing structure in traditional golf, the PDGA remains the single governing body of the sport, establishes the rules of play, and continues to manage and promote a single professional tour.

Today there is a compelling emphasis on bringing disc golf to young people and attracting more women to the sport. Each year, the PDGA awards grants to people who develop innovative ideas for growing the sport at the grassroots level. Women-only leagues and tournaments are developing all over the US in an effort to bring the game to more women. The National Collegiate Disc Golf Championships have taken hold and offer students from more than 60 colleges and universities in the US a way to compete against their contemporaries in a spirited setting. Most people profoundly involved in the sport believe the recreational side of disc golf offers the greatest opportunity for growth. Because of its beginner-friendly skill set, inexpensive start-up cost, and low environmental impact, the popularity of disc golf at all levels is clearly on the upswing.

Chapter 3

Disc Golf Course Design

The sport of disc golf is as much about the course as it is anything else, in large part because every one of the 6,000 or so disc golf courses in the world is unique. Tennis courts are the exact same dimensions whether you are playing in France or Fargo. Sure, there are different playing surfaces (grass, clay, hard court, and synthetic), and they do have some impact on shot execution, but the size of the court is a constant. The uniqueness of each disc golf course, in both its natural beauty and varied challenges, is a significant part of what makes playing disc golf a joyful pursuit. Courses serve different purposes. Some are designed to introduce new players to the game, and others are for championship tournament play. In this chapter, we describe the basic elements of a disc golf course and provide a thoughtful critique on what separates simply good courses from patently great ones.

Basic Elements of a Disc Golf Course

Disc golf courses differ significantly from traditional golf courses, but the terminology used to describe elements of both types is similar. Much like traditional golf, the differences between municipal/recreational and championship-caliber courses can be enormous. About half of all disc courses feature an 18-hole layout, and roughly 40 percent have a 9-hole layout. Disc golf courses are fundamentally much less expensive to build than traditional golf courses. An 18-hole disc golf course can be built for around $10,000 (the very best ones can cost up to $100,000), and the average maintenance cost per year is roughly a few hundred dollars. The average 18-hole traditional golf course frequently costs more than $10 million to construct, and the yearly maintenance costs can easily exceed $500,000.

In addition, disc golf courses require about one-third the land needed for traditional golf courses. Disc golf holes are much shorter in length than traditional golf holes, and are typically measured in feet rather than yards. Disc golf holes typically range from about 200 to 600 feet, although longer holes, some greater than 1,000 feet, are becoming fairly common.

Both disc and traditional golf courses have greens, fairways, and tee boxes (or tee pads, as they are often called in disc golf). Most traditional golf courses have three or four sets of tee boxes for juniors, women, men, and professionals that essentially consist of tee markers on nicely mown, level grass. Disc golf courses may have multiple tee pads on each hole that serve the same basic purpose. Tee pads may be constructed of concrete, rubber, artificial grass, dirt, mulch, or natural grass (the last type often called a natural pad). Concrete is the most popular choice; about 70 percent of players surveyed prefer concrete pads. The biggest issue with concrete pads is that the best shoes to wear for driving on concrete tee pads are not best for walking in the woods or on slippery grass. However, the durability and slip resistance of well-constructed concrete pads outweighs the minor footwear concern for many players.

An ideal-sized tee pad is around 5 feet wide by about 12 feet long. Rectangular pads are common, but trapezoids are better because they afford both right- and left-handed players the space to use different approach steps. Some pads are designed with two trapezoids to account for different approaches and different routes. The opposite photo illustrates this unique approach to tee pad design. In general, longer holes necessitate more steps on the tee pad while driving, and thus longer tee pads. The best disc golf courses often have multiple tee pads to add variety and combat erosion. Great course design requires artistry, but great tee pads are often the result of the labor of great disc golf clubs. Tee pad installation is fairly simple (much like building a small section of sidewalk), but it is quite labor intensive; therefore, the best pads are often built by groups.

As discussed, disc golf courses have numerous types of targets (also called baskets) instead of the flag/pin/hole combination used in traditional golf.

Examples of various types of targets can be seen in several of the photos used throughout this book. Many players still refer to targets as pins, but only absolute beginners call them goals or cages. The PDGA determines which targets are approved for tournament play, but some private courses have home-made targets constructed from wood, metal, bicycle rims, chain, wire, plastic tubing, or whatever the designer could find. Approved targets consist of metal poles with a basket assembly in which the disc comes to rest, and chains to slow down the disc as it approaches the pole in flight. Targets designed for tournament play typically have two or more sets of heavy-gauge chains designed to create a spiderweb effect to "catch" an approaching disc.

Every target manufacturer claims to have the best approved target, but the top models from each major manufacturer are basically the same. Some older target courses still utilize objects such as metal or wood poles that a player must hit to complete the hole. Of course, this can get tricky when a player appears to hit the target from a distance. Some people say that PDGA-approved targets "make a course," and we tend to agree with them.

In lieu of, or in addition to, multiple tee pads, disc golf courses may have multiple target placements. It is neither difficult nor expensive to install multiple metal sleeves and to simply move the target from one sleeve to another to create various target placements.

All traditional golf holes, including ones in wooded areas, have well-defined open areas of meticulously mown grass called fairways on which players attempt to land their balls. In disc golf, fairways range on a continuum from wide open to densely wooded. Open fairways may have few trees, nicely mown grass, or even lush farm fields. Some

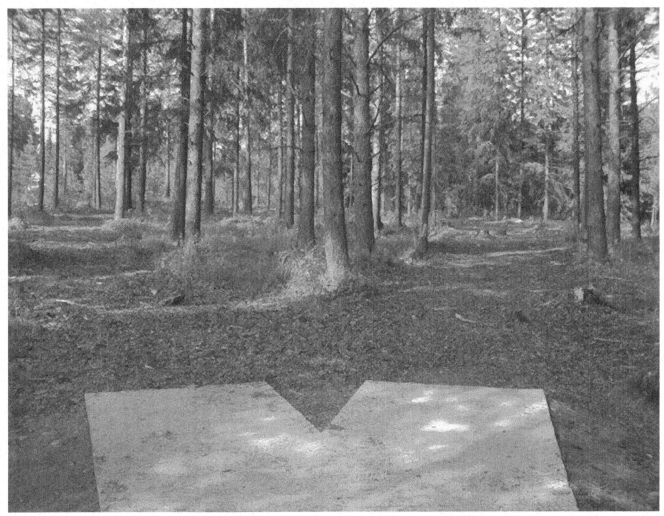

The tee pad on hole 12 at the Discgolf Terminalen in Västerbotten, Sweden. *Photo courtesy of dgcoursereview.com*

open disc golf fairways may even share space with traditional golf courses. During tournament play, yellow ropes can be used to delineate fairways and **out-of-bounds** (OB) areas on holes at the open end of the continuum.

In disc golf, partially or densely wooded holes are common. They typically feature much narrower and less-defined fairways than found on traditional golf holes and feature dirt or mulch walking paths. Gaps between trees and other hazards, called routes or **flyways**, delineate where a player's thrown disc should navigate to reach the green or landing area

in the fairway. The best holes may have multiple routes to give players options for reaching the green or landing area.

A disc golf green is essentially a landing area near the target on which players attempt to land their thrown discs in order to have a good chance of making a putt. Some greens are covered with mulch to help stop a thrown disc from bouncing or rolling away from the target, but others are entangled with tree roots that may cause your disc to take an ill-fated (or perhaps lucky) skip or **roll**. Greens with tree roots do little to curtail erosion and

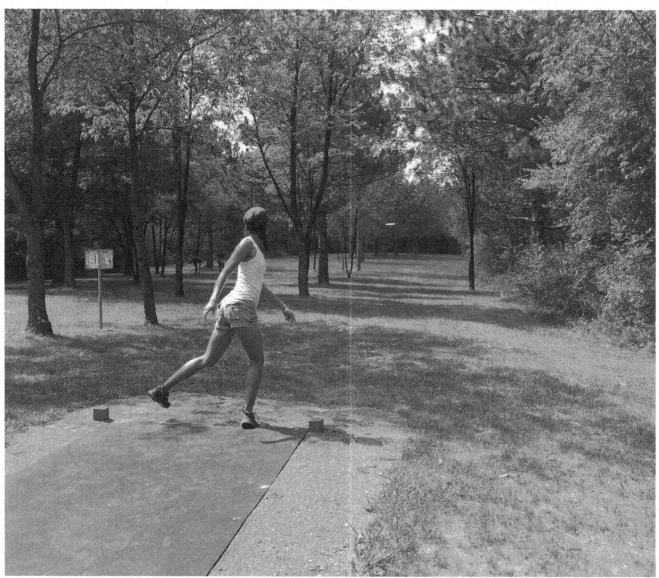

Melody King chooses the right route on hole 6 at Moraine State Park in Portersville, Pennsylvania. *Photo by Jerry Gotcher and courtesy of Innova Champion Discs*

are certainly much less desirable than those with mulch. Elevated or sloping greens are commonly found on disc golf courses to increase the challenge of landing a thrown disc near the target. Greens adjacent to ponds, lakes, and rivers may also add beauty and challenge to a hole. Targets protruding from rocks or tree stumps add a natural staging dimension to a green; elevated baskets are also fairly common. Some greens are built with landscaping timbers to create a dramatic landing area as well as to combat erosion.

What Makes a Great Disc Golf Course?

There are those people in the world who spend much of their time designing great disc golf courses. People like John Houck, Stan McDaniel, Chuck Kennedy, and Harold Duvall come to mind, but there are others. Course architects with vast experience know best what makes a great disc golf course, but as folks who live for playing great courses, we have our own horse in the race. As you might expect, there are thousands of good disc golf courses but precious few *great* ones. All the great courses have a few common characteristics; simply stated, they are beautiful, challenging, fair, and "safe" (minimize risk). A lot of people would add *fun* to this list, and we are fine with that. But in the end, we think if you are playing a beautiful and challenging course, having fun is up to you.

Beauty

We believe that truly great disc golf courses are, above all else, naturally beautiful. Beauty may be in the eye of the beholder, but some elements of beauty are universally accepted. In his book *Symmetry and Complexity: The Spirit and Beauty of Nonlinear Science*, Klaus Mainzer details how beauty and simplicity emerge from nonlinear, ever-evolving systems. To call Mainzer's work an easy read would be ludicrous, but you do not have to be a mathematician to wrap your head around the idea that order from chaos is everywhere and that art is not as unscientific as one might believe. Truly beautiful disc golf courses take advantage of natural elements in a way that makes players feel as though they are not merely rambling around a field or through the

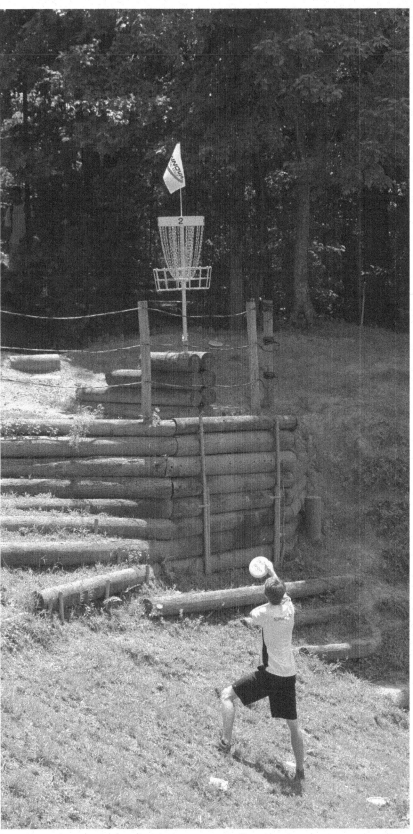

Will Schusterick putts on the nerve-racking, Stan McDaniel–designed hole 2 green at Renaissance Park in Charlotte, North Carolina. *Photo by Ryan Bumgarner*

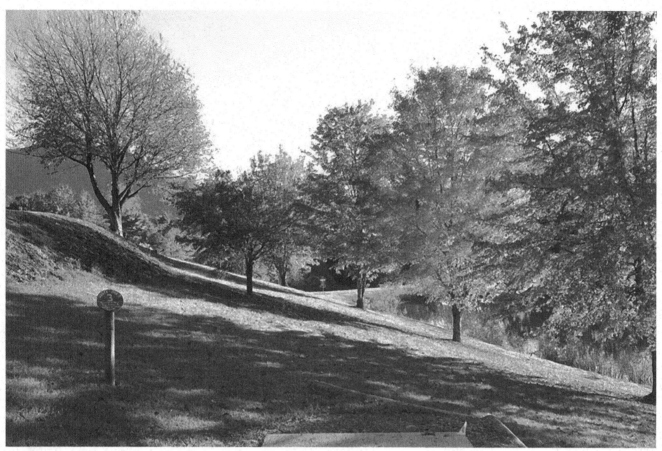

The view from the short tee pad on hole 3 of the Ashe County Disc Golf Course in Jefferson, North Carolina. *Photo by Todd Patoprsty and used with permission from Innova Champion Discs*

woods. These courses pose problems that are not answered by the same, simple solution over and over again. Also, truly beautiful courses tend to finish where they started, while the journey was filled with inevitable highs and lows.

The most beautiful courses possess all the diversity that natural elements have to offer. They have a variety of native grasses, trees, shrubs, flowering plants, and rock formations. Many of them also have water elements such as lakes, ponds, rivers, and streams. Courses designed in mountainous terrain are often rugged and technical, while those near coastal waters might be lush and/or marshy. Personally, we love scenic mountaintop vistas and dramatic elevation changes, but there are some stunning ocean-side courses with very little elevation change.

One of the most remote and naturally beautiful courses in the US is at Ashe County Park in West Jefferson, North Carolina, and was designed by Harold Duvall. The elevation changes are momentous and the scenic views are majestic.

Challenge

Designing great courses is as much science as artistry, and the science is based on the statistical likelihood of successfully executed throws. Designing challenging holes and courses is a dynamic and complex process. Ultimately *challenge* means the odds that a skilled player will successfully earn a par on a given hole, and for the entire course, fall somewhere between decent and pretty good. Par should be attainable but far from guaranteed. Earning a par on a given hole, and for the entire course, should be challenging to the average player. Longer holes will often have a different par for recreational and professional players. The par for the hole is typically posted on a sign next to the tee pad and indicated on the scorecard.

To estimate degree of challenge, course designers calculate the average score on a given hole by examining scores of many players of differing skill levels. This metric, common to traditional golf, is called the **stroke average**. For example, if a par-3 hole has a stroke average of 3.5, the hole is playing half a stroke (throw) over par. Ideally holes should have a stroke average around par. If a hole has a stroke average far above or below par, the hole might be far too challenging or simply not challenging enough. Stroke average is not the only measure of how challenging a hole is to the average player, but it is a quick and simple calculation.

The best course designers will also examine the percentages. Presume a given hole has a stroke average around par. However, on that same hole, more than 70 percent of players earn a **birdie**. How is that possible? Well, if the other 30 percent earn scores far above par, then it is likely that stroke average is not a good indicator of how the hole is playing. Collecting stroke averages and percentages is valuable but does not tell the whole story. To truly assess degree of challenge, great course designers may also examine issues that yield conflicting stroke averages and percentages, such as poorly placed tee pads and out-of-bounds delineations.

Challenge should be about rewarding excellent throws and not about simple risk-versus-reward. A hole could have reasonable metrics but still be considered what course designer John Houck calls a dumb hole. What makes a hole dumb? Challenging holes reward good throws, but dumb holes reward luck over skill, or offer little reward for good throws. Many dumb holes are simply the wrong distance—too long to yield many birdies or too short to yield many **bogeys**. Another type of dumb hole is called the poke-and-hope or throw-and-pray hole. If the only route through trees or other obstacles is extremely narrow, then the chance even an experienced disc golfer will execute a successful throw is so low that it can be called dumb luck. On densely wooded courses, dumb holes are far too common. If you are lucky enough to navigate your drive through the very narrowly spaced trees, you are almost guaranteed a par or birdie. If you do not, you are facing a bogey or worse. Of course, there is a gray area between luck and skill. As the saying goes, you make your own luck, and everyone has to play the same hole.

In order for a hole and an entire course to be challenging for players of all levels—which is very tough to pull off—multiple tee pads and target placements are vital. On great courses, multiple tee pads do more than simply add distance to the hole. They create different routes and thus encourage players to choose different types of drives from the tee pad. Ideally, mutliple targets should not simply add distance; they should define unique greens in which a player attempts to land his or her disc and thus present unique challenges.

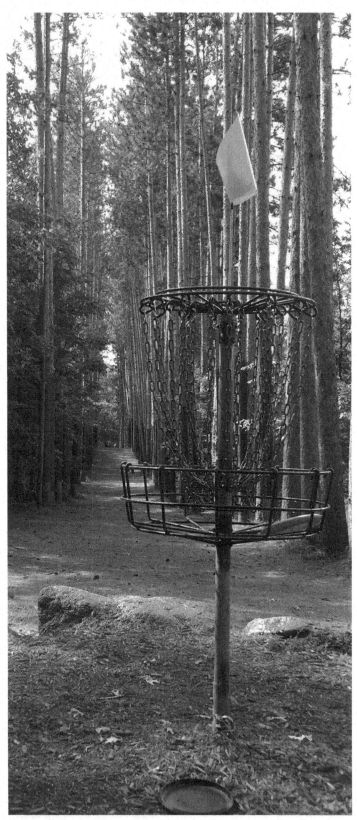

A look back down the tight fairway on the famous hole 4 on the Blue Ribbon Pines Disc Golf Course in East Bethel, Minnesota. *Photo courtesy of PDGA Media*

Also, we believe—as Houck and others do as well—that great disc golf courses should more closely resemble great traditional golf courses than miniature golf courses. As such, a truly great disc golf course has a blend of par-3, par-4, and par-5 holes. Longer holes are logically more difficult, but a great par-4 or par-5 hole should reward accuracy and not just distance. Making a hole longer, and thus increasing its stroke average, does not make it better. The best long holes require a player to navigate various routes and execute two or more good throws to earn par. Some of our favorite holes offer the unique challenges that elevation changes afford and/or give players the opportunity to throw over a natural body of water. After all, changes in elevation and water hazards often require both accuracy and distance control.

We feel artificial out-of-bounds areas can be unsightly and frustrating. Increasing the level of challenge by adding artificial OB to an open course is, at times, a necessary evil, but the very best courses do not need to sacrifice beauty for challenge. Houck described the psychological impact of artificial OB best: "When you realize your disc is in the water, your first thought is typically, *I hope I can find it.* If your disc comes to rest in a painted or roped-off OB area, your first response is, *Are you kidding me? I can't throw from here?*"

Challenge does not equate to silliness. Holes with weird target placements make us feel like we are playing a miniature golf course with spinning windmills and plaster frogs. Targets swinging on ropes, half-buried

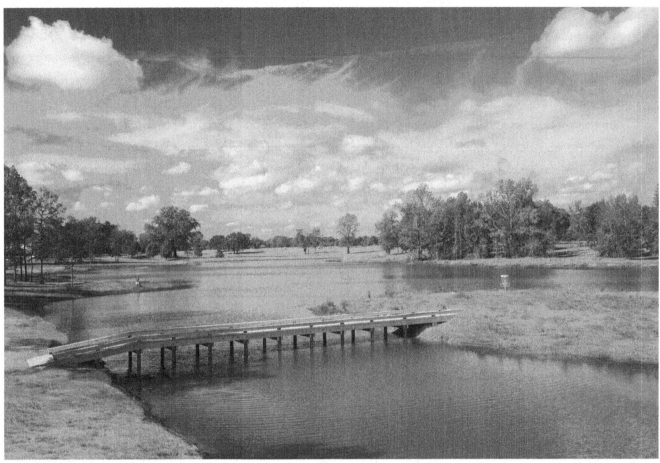

The challenging hole 7 on the John Houck–designed Lakeside course at Selah Ranch in Talco, Texas. Houck (at left center) is standing at the ideal spot for an approach throw to the spectacular island green. *Photo courtesy of Jumping Rocks Photography*

underground, or hidden in a maze of wood or brush just seem silly to us. Puerile, tacky, and fluky holes that reward luck over skill are often called **clown holes**. Elevated targets are fine, as long as nearly all players can reach into the target to retrieve their disc without climbing a ladder. Of course, when designing a course that will be used exclusively by children, silly is just fine as long as fairness is paramount. Fairness and safety should never be sacrificed in an attempt to make a hole challenging. There are ways to design a disc golf course that is both challenging and fair without adding distance, planting hundreds of trees, or creating a man-made body of water.

Fairness

Fairness is an important attribute found in all great disc golf courses. As a general rule, a great 18-hole course should have about six holes on which players must throw straight off the tee pad, six on which they must shape their drive right, and six on which they must shape their drive left. The 6-6-6 rule is just a guide, and each course designer has his or her own idea of what constitutes a fair and balanced course. As such, it is acceptable for a course to have only three or four drives that must be thrown straight to reach a landing area or green. Longer holes should require a combination of straight and shaped throws. For example, a par-4 hole may require a straight drive to land on the fairway, then a left-to-right throw to land on the green.

Some folks feel that fairness to left- and right-handed players is important, as it is in traditional golf, but we do not believe it is a major issue in disc golf. After all, regardless of your "handedness," you may throw using a backhand or forehand style. Using different throwing styles enables a player to throw a disc that flies either left to right or right to left. Still, the prevailing wisdom in course design is that there needs to be a balance between lefty and righty shots. Players should be able to throw both backhands and forehands when needed, but to expect recreational players to throw both styles equally well is too arduous a task.

Truly great courses are both challenging and fair in that they provide an honest test of a player's skills. Great courses are designed to ensure four things: 1) that players who can throw both far and with accuracy have the greatest advantage, 2) that players who can throw far will have the opportunity to gain a few strokes on a few of the holes, 3) that players who throw accurately will have an opportunity to gain a few strokes on a few of the holes, and 4) that players who demonstrate the most skillful performance will earn the best scores. The very best courses in the world are composed of mostly great holes. The thousands of *good* courses in the world typically have a few great holes, a few holes that offer little challenge to skilled players, and a few holes that are just plain dumb.

Safety

Speaking of dumb, courses that pose a serious threat to the safety of players and other users are the dumbest of all. Safety might seem like an obvious component, but as the number of courses has skyrocketed, the potential for conflict between a facility and its users has increased as well. Recreational parks and school grounds are tempting places to build courses because they expose the sport to many people of all ages and abilities; however, these areas are also the most prone to risk. While no disc golf course or any other sports venue is 100 percent safe, many of the potentially problematic courses are located at recreational parks and on school property.

Recreational park directors and school administrators often work with limited budgets, and the allure of an inexpensive facility is tempting for some, often at a detriment to safety. Sometimes a disc golfer with little to no experience in course design offers to build a course at no charge, and the results can be unsatisfactory for both the players and the public. As the number of courses continues to grow, inexperienced designers may sacrifice more responsible choices to produce more challenging play (or to cut financial corners). Some course designers are egocentric by nature and may not ask for assistance avoiding potential hazards. Many players appreciate great courses and realize that paying for a top designer is worth the price. When players have a voice in the development of a course, they should do their best to convince the people in charge to consider using the best available architect.

All disc golf courses (even those that are not particularly beautiful, challenging, or fair) should have adequate signage warning other facility users (in the case of courses in public parks) of the risk of flying discs and educating players on their personal responsibilities.

Conclusion

As more disc golf courses are built, the truly beautiful, challenging, fair, and safe ones will undoubtedly stand out. Fortunately, there are great courses located all over the US and the world in places like Burlington, Kentucky; Conifer, Colorado; Leicester, Massachusetts; Newtown, Pennsylvania; Shelby, Michigan; and Stockholm, Sweden.

When you are searching for the next great course to play, we recommend using two pieces of technology. One, install the PDGA app on your cell phone. You can easily search the database for courses near your current location, save information about your favorite courses, and even get driving directions. You will not find any super-secret private courses in this database, but it is a good starting point. Two, check out Disc Golf Course Review at dgcoursereview.com. There, you will find course data, user-submitted reviews, and photos of more than 4,000 courses.

The thousands of unique courses available for all to play are what make disc golf an exciting and challenging lifetime sport. Finding the very best courses is not as much of a challenge as it once was, but playing the ones on your bucket list is still a thrilling experience. Friendly competition, trying out new equipment, and improving on your game all help make disc golf an addictive outdoor pursuit, but the courses themselves are the most important ingredient. Great disc golf courses are intriguing, convoluted puzzles for players to solve, and the best courses immerse players in a natural, wondrous artist's canvas.

Chapter 4

Rules and Etiquette Every Player Should Know

Much like its traditional golf sibling, disc golf is a game of rules, and there are a lot of them. The Professional Disc Golf Association (PDGA) is the national and international governing body of the sport, and establishes the rules and competition standards. *Official Rules of Disc Golf* and *Competition Manual for Disc Golf Events* are published separately by the PDGA. As its title indicates, the latter contains guidelines and special rules used in tournament play. Of course, you do not need to know every rule to enjoy playing a casual round of disc golf, but there are some fundamental rules that every player should know and follow to make playing an enjoyable experience for everyone.

Uber-competitive disc golfers who thrive on tournament play should know the rules better than casual players, which is why the PDGA requires players to pass a rules examination before they can play in Majors and National Tour events. Rarely is there a certified official following a group around the course, except perhaps during major tournaments. Instead, when questions arise, getting a group consensus in a timely manner is standard protocol. Some people are sticklers for the rules and like to refer to the official rule book as often as they can.

During both casual rounds and tournament play, we judiciously abide by the rules of disc golf—but with a relaxed attitude. To be honest, we play by the rules out of habit more than to further something as lofty as honor, pride, or respect. If a player does not abide by a particular rule during play, we ask the other group members if they noticed the same infraction. If they did, we try to point out the rule to the offending player in a very non-abrasive way. Nothing says *newbie* more than not playing by the rules.

Discs Used During Play

Technically, you must use a disc approved for tournament play by the PDGA. With more than 600 approved discs available, that is not a major issue. You may not use a disc that is cracked or punctured, but using a **seasoned disc** that you sanded a bit is acceptable. You may use a disc designed primarily for throw-and-catch, such as the Discraft Ultra-Star. The Aerobie flying ring (essentially a wide rim with no center section) is not legal for play. Carrying an illegal disc is not a punishable offense; you must throw it for there to be a penalty. If you choose to throw an illegal disc, the consequence is two **penalty throws** without a warning if a player in your group calls you on it.

Most players write their name and phone number on the bottom of each of their discs. Technically, you must have a distinguishing mark on your discs during tournament play, but from a practical standpoint, you are more likely to get a lost disc back if you have your name and number on it. Most players make it a point to return lost discs to their rightful owners, whenever possible. This common courtesy is called into question each semester that we teach beginning disc golf. Some of our students are in awe that folks actually try to return lost discs to their owners. "What if I spend an hour wading in the pond for my disc and find someone else's disc?" someone inevitably asks. We tell them that if they find one of our discs, we will give them a few dollars for their effort. There is some debate as to when a lost disc becomes the property of someone else. Many used sporting goods stores have shelves of discs with names on the bottom. Most players are so grateful to get their disc back, the "finder's fee" is worth the paltry expense.

Score-Related Terms

Simply stated, par on any given hole is the number of throws (or strokes) an experienced player is expected to need to complete the hole. In disc golf, par-3 holes are most frequent. In fact, on many courses all the holes are par-3. Par-4s and par-5s are becoming more common on disc golf courses, and a lot of people think that is a good idea. If you add all the pars for each hole together, then you get the par for the entire course. A lot of 18-hole courses are par-54 (or darn close), so when doing quick math in our heads to calculate our score, we use 54 as a starting point. Par is a simple, quantifiable entity, but it can represent much more. It can be puzzling, seductive, elusive, and sometimes seemingly unattainable. But par is universal. If martians landed their flying saucer on a disc golf course, they would have to play against par just as any human being would. As silly as it sounds, that seems pretty cool to us.

A birdie is one throw less than par. For example, on a par-3 hole a birdie is a score of 2, or a **deuce**, as it is often called. Birdies are good, and we all want to get them. Two throws under par—such as a score of 2 on a par-4 hole—is called an **eagle**. A score of 2 on a par-5 hole is called a **double eagle**. Eagles and double eagles are rare and beautiful birds. A bogey is one throw over par. For example, on a par-4 hole, a bogey is a score of 5. Bogeys are bad, and nobody wants to get one. But a bogey is better than a **double bogey** (two throws over par) or a triple bogey (three throws over par). Some players like to call a double bogey on a par-3 hole a fistful or handful, and a triple bogey on a par-5 hole a snowman.

If a player takes only one throw to complete the hole, then he has earned a hole in one or ace, as it is most often called. In our opinion, aces are one of the best aspects of playing disc golf. They occur much more frequently than in traditional golf, because many disc golf holes are par-3 and many of those holes are realistically "aceable." Some players claim to have hundreds of career aces, while some people who have been playing for years have none. When someone gets an ace, it is almost always cause for boisterous celebration. It is customary for each person witnessing an ace to sign the thrown disc, and for that reason it is good to keep a permanent marker in your bag, just in case. Most players have witnesses sign the bottom of the disc and put the disc right back in their bag, ready for another ace.

Most weekly club events have ace pools, in which each player has the option of putting a dollar or two in the pot each week. When someone hits an ace, that person gets the pot. These pots of money often grow week after week, and it is not unusual to see ace pots of hundreds of dollars. We have even heard of people driving hundreds of miles to weekly club events because of large ace pots.

Teeing Off

A player must tee off from the tee pad or a designated tee area. As the disc is released from your throwing hand, you must have one foot on the pad or behind a line designated by tee markers. If you are teeing off with proper driving form, you will firmly plant a foot on the tee pad, and your momentum will likely cause your non-plant foot to land near or beyond the edge of the tee pad. You may start with one or both feet off the tee pad as long as your plant foot ends up on the pad when you release the disc. While teeing off, you do not have to demonstrate balance after you release the disc.

Order of Play

Which player tees off from the first tee? Whoever is listed on the scorecard first. Who determines that? During tournament play, the **tournament director**

(often called the TD) usually does. During casual play, it does not really matter that much. Of course, local clubs have their own customs. Regardless of when you tee off, you should never throw when players, spectators, or other facility users are within range. If it is a **blind throw**, send the player teeing off last down the fairway to act as spotter to make sure the course is clear.

This next rule might be the most important rule in disc golf because of the safety aspect. After each player throws from the tee box, the player farthest from the target, called the **away player**, throws first. This greatly reduces the chances that a player will get whacked in the head with a disc, assuming you are not advancing down the fairway ahead of the group. Often, two throws come to rest nearly equidistant from the target. When this happens, the player who is closer to the target may throw first if both players contend that it is okay to do so. Sometimes serious discussions take place when two or more competing players are putting from approximately the same distance. It happens occasionally when a player feels he is closer to the target (or in) and wants to see if a competitor (who he/she thinks is out) makes his/her putt. During casual play, some folks like to play **ready golf**, which allows for players to putt or throw out of order (with courtesy) to speed up the pace of the game.

The scores on the preceding hole determine the teeing order on the following hole, with the lowest score throwing first, and so on. If the preceding hole had a tie, the scores are to be counted back until the order is determined. Ties seem to happen more often than not, and if you are keeping the scorecard for the group, this is a good time to ask for help if needed. It is common to play with people who are good at keeping score but can never get the order exactly right.

Keeping Score

As discussed earlier, the goal is to complete each hole, and ultimately the course, in the fewest number of throws. This is one of those less-is-better kinds of scenarios in life, and the math could not be easier. You simply write down the number of throws it took you to finish each hole, including any penalty strokes, then add the number of throws from each of the holes together at the end of the round to come up with your total number of throws for the round.

Much like in traditional golf, playing in foursomes is common in disc golf. Keeping a scorecard for a group of players can be a bit complicated, but if you follow some pretty simple steps, you can avoid arguments over scoring. First, we cannot think of a situation when a player would write his/her scores relative to par rather than the actual number of throws in the little boxes on a scorecard. If it takes you four throws to complete a hole, do not get creative; simply write the number *4* in the box. If your disc went out-of-bounds at some point during play on the hole, it is customary to circle the number. During tournament play, each group keeps one official scorecard and submits it to the tournament director after the round.

Some rules may vary by tournament, but a good practice is that the player who tees off first keeps the group scorecard for four or so holes and then passes it on to the next person listed on the scorecard. In this way, at the end of the round, each person had an opportunity to keep score for the group. Of course, in addition to a group scorecard, a player may keep his or her own scorecard.

Players have differing opinions on keeping a scorecard during a round, and that is fine, but we do not think a person can go wrong with the following strategy. First, stand or sit close enough for everyone to clearly hear you. Next, announce your score on the previous hole loud enough for everyone to hear by saying something like, "That was hole 7. I got a 4." Then ask each person in succession what they scored, announce each person's score to the group, then write each number in the corresponding box on the card. Do this for every hole, even if it was obvious what a player scored. Nobody minds repeating they earned a score of 2 on a hole, and it gives folks an opportunity to say something like "Nice deuce, dude!" It may be a little uncomfortable when someone cards an 8, but there is just no way around it. If you follow this protocol, it is very clear what each person scored on the previous hole. Do not forget to then announce the teeing order, and do not be afraid to ask for help from the group to get the teeing order correct.

Marking the Lie

After each throw, a player must leave his or her disc where it came to rest until the lie is established, by placing a mini marker disc on the ground between the target and the disc. Technically, the marker should be touching the thrown disc, but if a player places it a few millimeters in front of the thrown disc, that player is not likely to catch any flak. Most of the time, players can choose to use the thrown disc to mark their lie, but they must be careful not to move it. A player must use a marker disc when repositioning a lie. This occurs most often when a player's thrown disc comes to rest out-of-bounds. Flipping your disc as it lies on the ground in lieu of marking it is not legal in tournament play but is fine if you are playing a casual round.

It is fair to say that most players use a mini marker disc most of the time. If given the option, when would a player not want to get eight or so inches closer to the target? Well, when you are pretty far away from the target, it is easier to use your thrown disc to mark the lie. If a player's disc comes to rest up against a tree or other obstacle, players may choose not to use a marker disc so they have a better angle to the target. This occurs more often than you might think on tight, wooded courses.

One rule often overlooked by novice players concerns taking relief. If your disc comes to rest in bounds but within one meter of an out-of-bounds line, the lie may be relocated to any point on a one-meter line that extends perpendicular from the nearest point of the out-of-bounds line, and passes through the center of the thrown disc. It is important to note this holds true even if the direction takes the lie closer to the target. So if your disc comes to rest up against a fence or a few feet from a lake, you can take a meter of relief to establish a legal **stance**. Many beginners either forget this rule or are not aware of it. Again, when in doubt, ask the group if taking relief is appropriate.

Legal Stance

Of all the calls made by players on other players, the ones called most often are stance violations. Asking other players in your group if they think your stance is legal is typically okay, but even novices should know where they can stand. Basically players have to stand either behind their disc as it lies on the ground or behind a marker disc. It sounds pretty simple, but the devil is in the details.

Usually a player's throwing stance is simply standing on two feet. Occasionally players may have one foot and one knee on the ground, or both knees if their lie is poor, such as when their disc comes to rest under some foliage. Speaking of foliage, a player cannot break tree branches or hold them out of the way with his or her non-throwing hand in an attempt to get a clearer shot to the target. If players accidentally step on a few tall weeds in an attempt to place their marker discs, that is acceptable, but they cannot intentionally trample foliage to create a line of sight or tunnel through which to throw. Nor can players touch a tree branch or obstacle to improve their line of sight or maintain balance. Remember to keep your hands, feet, and backside off foliage and obstacles.

For a stance to be considered legal, both feet or supporting points must be in bounds, and one foot or supporting point must be within 30 centimeters directly behind the marker disc. Novice players often overlook the operative word here: *directly*. Equally as important, your other foot or supporting point cannot be placed any closer to the target than the marker disc. Most of the time you simply place a foot a few inches behind the marker disc, draw an imaginary line from the marker disc to the target, and then draw another imaginary line that is roughly perpendicular to that line to establish a legal stance. It sounds complicated, but it only takes a few seconds. You cannot step on the marker disc as you are throwing, so always try to give yourself a few inches to spare.

10-Meter Rule

Any throw from within 10 meters (about 33 feet) or less, as measured from the rear of the marker disc to the base of the hole, is considered a putt. If a player's **follow-through** after a putt causes him or her to make any supporting point (like a foot or hand) contact the ground closer to the hole than the rear edge of the marker disc, that player has committed a stance violation. A player must demonstrate full control of balance before advancing toward the hole. The penalty (if two or more players in the group call you on it) is a verbal warning for the first offense. Subsequent violations in the same round result in a one-throw penalty for each infraction. Stance violations also result in a mandatory re-throw. If you are guilty of a stance violation and miss your putt, good luck getting two players to call you on it, thus giving you another chance to make the putt. Also, you cannot call a stance violation on yourself.

Stepping past the marker disc after you release the disc is okay if your marker is 10 meters or more from the target. If you are 10 meters or greater from the target, you may leap from behind your marker and let your momentum cause you to land somewhere in front of your marker. In fact, you can land flat on your face if you choose. This is called a **jump putt**, although it is technically not a putt at all, given it is from more than 10 meters away. One of the most asked questions by fellow competitors during a disc golf round is, "Am I 10 meters or more from the target?" But since that takes too long to say, a lot of folks just ask, "Am I 30 out?"

Excessive Time

You have a maximum of 30 seconds to throw once the course is clear after the previous player has thrown and after you have had a reasonable amount of time to arrive at your disc. If other players are in your throwing range, you are not on the clock. Don't throw if there is a chance you are putting other players, spectators, or other facility users in danger. Most often, excessive time is not a major issue. In windy conditions it is okay to wait for a calm period; just be aware that you are on the clock. While putting, experienced players tend to take most of their allotted time. Touring professionals seem to take forever.

Holing Out

A hole is completed when a player releases the disc and it comes to rest in the lower basket assembly of a disc golf target or when it is supported by the chains. (The disc may be additionally supported by the pole.) Discs that land on the very top section of the target are not considered holed out. If your disc comes to rest on top, you are faced with the easiest putt on the course. Simply set your marker disc a few inches from the base of the target and drop your disc in the basket assembly as your friends chuckle. Just don't rest your wrist or elbow on the basket assembly while you drop in your putt.

If your disc manages to enter the target from the top section (which can only realistically be done on certain styles of targets), or it somehow enters the target through the metal grating on the lower basket assembly, you have not successfully holed out. Of course, if nobody sees it happen, then nobody will ever know. If an official or two or more players in the group see it happen, then it is not

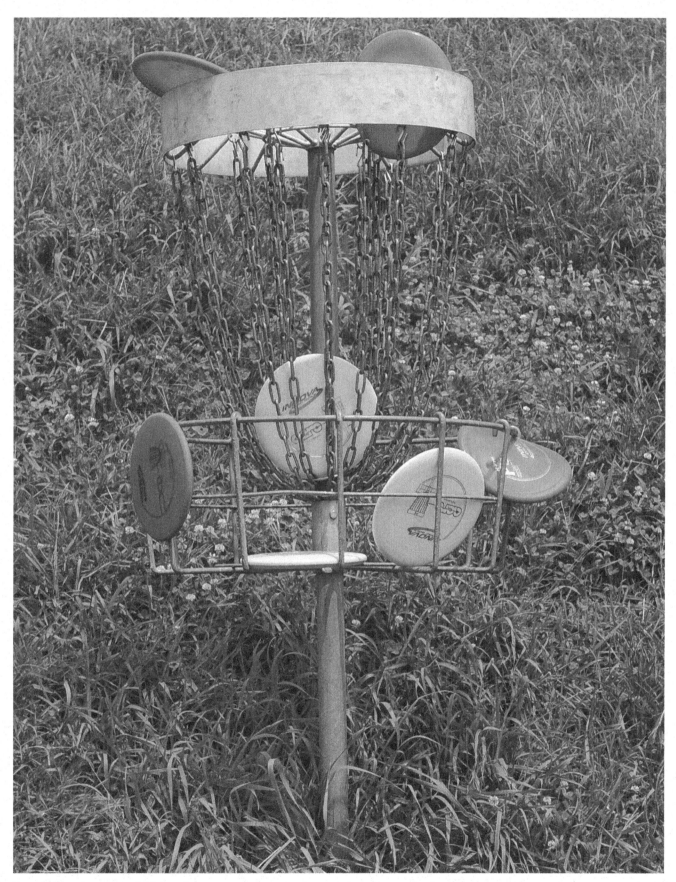

Successful and unsuccessful hole-outs. *Photo by Cyndy Caravelis*

considered holed out. The photo on page 55 depicts successful and unsuccessful hole-outs. The lower four discs are successful hole-outs, but the upper discs are not.

After you hole out, it is customary to remove your disc from the target before others attempt to hole out. You should at least ask, "Do you want me to clear that?" If you do not, other players may ask, "Can you clear that for me?" This often happens when your disc is supported by the chains or partially supported by the pole and the basket assembly (sometimes called a trampoline), as players fear their discs will bounce off your disc. If you have any doubt, pull it out. If there are players on the hole behind you, do not forget to yell something like "Hole 10 is clear!" to let them know the hole is ready for play.

Out-of-Bounds

If your disc lands out-of-bounds, you are in a quandary. You may not throw from your lie even if you can somehow establish a legal stance. A disc is considered out-of-bounds when it comes to rest and it is clearly and completely surrounded by the out-of-bounds area. Water, unless it is deemed **casual water** (such as puddles and marshy areas), is almost always considered out-of-bounds. Group debate may ensue if a disc is mostly in the water but is touching a small blade of grass in bounds. During tournament play, tournament directors determine what is out-of-bounds before play begins. When playing a casual round, consult the locals for the course rules. As a default assumption, take for granted that water, concrete, and asphalt are always out-of-bounds.

If your disc comes to rest out-of-bounds, you must take one penalty throw, but you do have a

few choices when it comes to where to play your next shot. You can play it from your previous lie, a designated drop zone, or from a lie that is up to one meter away from and perpendicular to the point where the disc last crossed into out-of-bounds, even if the direction takes the lie closer to the target. It is important to know this rule, because situations arise that make one choice advantageous over the others. We brainstormed about 100 different scenarios but settled on two common ones to illustrate our point.

Imagine you are playing a 300-foot par-3 hole. Your drive hits the ground, takes a bad bounce, and then comes to rest in a creek about 10 feet from the target, but there is no designated drop zone. You can opt to drive again from the tee pad, but you will be essentially throwing your third shot because of the penalty throw. To earn your par, you will have to make a tough 300-foot throw that would be considered an ace if it was not for that darn out-of-bounds penalty. Instead, put your marker disc one meter from where your thrown disc was last in bounds, and make your 10-foot putt this time. It took you two throws to complete the hole, plus one penalty throw, equaling three throws on the scorecard. Go ahead and circle the number 3 on the scorecard, indicating you were out-of-bounds on that particular hole, and pat yourself on the back because you saved par.

Second, suppose you have a severely uphill 20-foot putt for a score of 2 and a birdie. You bounce your disc off the top of the target, it rolls 50 feet down the very hill you are standing on, and comes to rest out-of-bounds. You could mark the disc where it went out-of-bounds and try a difficult, uphill 50-foot putt. Instead, stand back over your marker disc (if you moved it, you need group consensus as to where it was), and attempt your 20-foot putt again. You make it, so it takes you three throws to complete the hole plus one penalty throw for a circle-four. Pat yourself on the back for knowing the rule and that 50 feet is longer than 20.

Lost Discs

If you lose a thrown disc, you have three minutes to find it. The three-minute countdown does not start until you arrive at the spot where it was last seen, and when two players (or an official) let you know you are on the clock. All the players in the group are supposed to help you look for a lost disc if you ask them to do so. That does not mean players have to put themselves at physical risk searching for another player's lost disc. A player who is sensitive to poison ivy, for example, is not obligated to trounce through it in an effort to find a disc. Making an effort in this case is more important than trying to follow the rule judiciously, and three minutes often translates to five or more.

A lost disc means you must add a penalty throw to your score for that hole. If it was a tee shot, you must re-tee even if it means an exhausting sojourn up a long, steep hill to the tee pad. If your throw was not made from the tee, the group determines where you last threw from, and you must place your mini marker at that spot. Most bodies of water that pose a threat to thrown discs have a designated drop zone. In any event, you must count the original throw plus a penalty throw on your scorecard.

Mandatories

A **mandatory** (often called a mando) constrains the route a thrown or rolled disc may take

to the target. A thrown disc must pass to the designated side of the mandatory before the hole is completed. Mandos are often indicated by an arrow or a yellow marking. For example, if your disc must pass to the left of a large tree, an arrow pointing to the left might be affixed to the tree. The mandatory line is a straight line through the mandatory, perpendicular to the line from the tee to the mandatory. Double mandos dictate your disc must pass to the right of one object and to the left of another, which oftentimes means between two trees. Triple mandos are not as common and often have a vertical component. For example, your thrown disc must pass between two trees and under a wooden sign joining the trees.

If your disc completely misses the mandatory, you will be assessed one penalty throw and you must re-tee or throw from a designated drop zone. If there is no drop zone, you must mark your lie within five meters of the mandatory object and one meter behind the mandatory line that extends from the correct side of the mandatory. If your disc hits a mandatory tree or object (which is pretty common), then you have to hope for a good kick. If it kicks deep and to the correct side, you made the mandatory. If it kicks backward, your next throw must make the mandatory. If it kicks to the incorrect side and comes to rest past the tree enough that it crosses the mandatory line, you missed the mandatory.

Mandos are often used in course design for a couple reasons. One reason is to discourage players from throwing close to or over dangerous areas. For example, your thrown disc might have to pass left of a light pole to discourage you from throwing over a parking lot located to the right side of the light pole. Mandos are also used to make holes more challenging. Personally, we dislike most mandos. Ideally, a disc golf hole should be both far enough from dangerous areas and challenging enough that there is no need for a mandatory. But in some cases mandos are a necessary evil.

Provisional Throws

Provisional throws (often called provos) are additional throws that are not added to a player's score if they are not ultimately used in completion of the hole. Players must announce they are throwing a provisional disc before they throw, but they may throw one at any time. Provisional throws are most often used when there is a better-than-average chance a player's disc is lost or out-of-bounds. This saves the time it would take for a player to re-tee or re-throw from the previous lie. Provisional throws can get complicated, particularly when you are playing a doubles event without a partner (more on that later) and have the option of using a mulligan.

The rules do not specifically state that players must use their provisional throw if their initial throw is out-of-bounds, nor do they indicate players must use their initial throw if a disc that was once thought to be lost is found. However, a provisional throw may not be subsequently declared to be an optional re-throw. We will illustrate some interesting real-life examples of provisional throws that we have witnessed. If you have been playing disc golf a while then you may have witnessed more peculiar examples.

Eric is playing a par-3 hole. His tee shot goes horribly awry and the group agrees there is a good chance it is hopelessly lost in the woods. Eric suggests that he throw a provisional, and the group

nods in agreement. His re-teed throw comes to rest 50 feet from the target. Much to the group's surprise, someone finds Eric's disc, which had come to rest in a thick grove of trees about 90 feet from the target. Eric wants to play from where his provisional throw lies, because he would have an easy 15-foot putt for a par, but he must play from where his original throw came to rest. It takes him two throws to clear the grove of trees and one impressive putt from 30 feet to card a bogey-4. Eric is not happy, but he understands that we all play by the same rules.

Andrew's second shot on a par-4 hole is just more than 100 feet from the target, and he must throw over a pond. After he throws, the group sees his disc skip in bounds about 10 feet from the basket and roll toward a creek. Andrew suggests he throw a provisional disc in case his disc rolled out-of-bounds. The group proposes that he does not, because it will not likely speed up play, but they concede to his wishes and tell him to let it fly. His provisional throw clears both the pond and creek and then comes to rest about 60 feet from the target. As the group approaches the target, they see that his original throw is indeed out-of-bounds and that it was last in bounds about 15 feet from the target. Andrew wants to play from where his original throw was last in bounds, but he must play from where his provisional throw came to rest. Frustrated that he chose to throw a provisional, it takes him three throws to hole out, and he cards a bogey-5.

Basic Etiquette

Not knowing and abiding by the most basic rules and etiquette, even during casual rounds, is not much fun for anyone. In disc golf, playing casual rounds might mean a player does not care much about his or her score, and that is just fine. But unless you are an absolute beginner, knowing and abiding by the basic rules and universal etiquette should be routine. Typically, discourteous behavior is easily recognized and often results in a courtesy warning from a group member. A second offense can result in a penalty throw if two or more players in your group (or any group) call you on it. Each subsequent courtesy violation results in a penalty throw. Repeated or excessive courtesy violations may result in disqualification. Etiquette is as much about what to do as it is about what *not* to do.

Most discourteous behavior falls into three general categories: 1) distracting another player while he or she is throwing, 2) acting like an imbecile, or 3) disgracing the course. Discourteous behavior includes: shouting, cursing, throwing out of turn, throwing or kicking golf bags, throwing minis, blowing smoke in the direction of other players, fiddling with discs while others are throwing, littering, destroying vegetation, and advancing on the fairway beyond the away player.

You should make every effort to avoid talking, moving around, or standing in the line of sight of a player while throwing, either on the tee on in the fairway. Players who habitually stand in other players' peripheral vision can drive them crazy. When possible, stand behind the player who is throwing. We prefer to stand behind a tree when standing behind the thrower is not feasible. Either way, you should always be still and quiet.

Writing or carving graffiti on benches, targets, or trees is juvenile and disgraceful. Littering, destroying course property, and obliterating vegetation are all serious offenses, and you should

never do them…period. Between rounds of a tournament, a professional player once grew tired of hitting the same tree limb with his discs, and thus he decided to climb a ladder and cut it down. He was caught, disqualified from the tournament, and suspended from playing in PDGA sanctioned tournaments for one year. The PDGA maintains a list of suspended players. Although you will not find the specific offenses listed by the suspended players' names, a few of these suspensions are a result of onetime excessive courtesy violations such as excessive swearing and alcohol/drug use during tournament rounds.

There is some etiquette you may not find in a rule book, such as protocol that speeds up the pace of play. For example, immediately after every person in the group has teed off, if you are clearly the away player (perhaps because you smacked your drive into the tree closest to the tee pad), you should grab your bag and try to be the first person advancing down the fairway. After all, since you will be the away player, everyone will be standing behind you while they wait for you to throw. Standing by your bag and fiddling with your discs (or chalk bag, scorecard, etc.) while everyone marches down the fairway may be annoying to others in the group.

Some players like to talk to their discs. That may sound strange, but the non-talkers might be the minority. Our colleague Chris Tuten always makes us laugh when he makes statements like "Flex a little, honey" as his disc is in flight. We recommend avoiding talking too much about the flight of another player's thrown disc. Many a disc golfer has said "Nice!" while another player's disc is taking a seemingly perfect route to the target, only for it to take a bad skip and end up in a creek.

Some people even make rude statements like "Don't nice my disc!" In general, we avoid **"nicing"** a player's disc until it completely comes to rest. Our friend Nate Kellar is one of the best at delivering witty, timely one-worders like "dirty" and "useful." Of course, proper etiquette during casual rounds may be different than during tournament rounds. While playing tournament rounds, it is best to say very little.

There are other distractions during play that can diminish the playing experience. They include but are not limited to letting your dog roam the course, drinking alcohol in excess during play, listening to music, and spinning your disc in your hand while others are throwing. Our personal pet peeve entails players listening to music using headphones/earbuds during play. During casual rounds, using headphones is a way to avoid being social (which is your choice), but there are times when rule interpretations arise, and we hate it when the group has to wait for a player to remove his or her headphones to join the conversation. The official rules permit headphone use during tournament play.

Part II

The Science of the Game

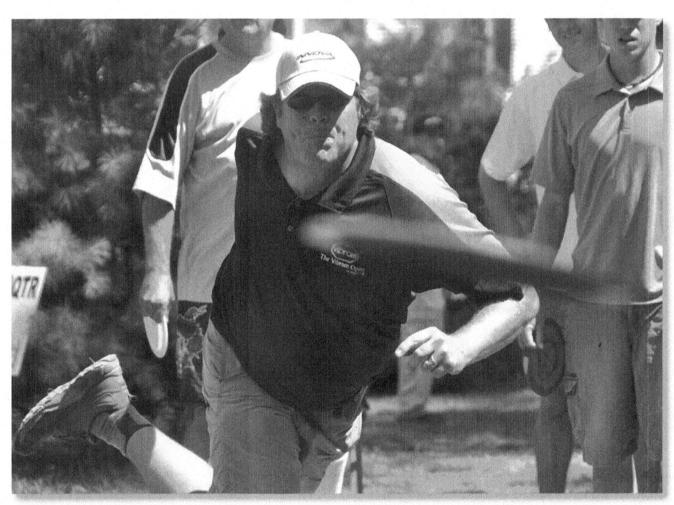

Jay "Yeti" Reading rips a backhand drive. *Photo by Eino Ansio and courtesy of Innova Champion Discs.*

Mental Training

Many people refer to both traditional golf and disc golf as mental games. Playing disc golf requires myriad physical skills, but without an effective mental game, you will never be able to consistently perform at or near your peak. A lot of people like to use the term *muscle memory*, but muscles do not have the capability to store memories. Your memories only reside in your brain. Even if you devote countless hours to physically practicing skills, your muscles will not remember anything. Your mind controls your muscles, and if it is not functioning optimally, your muscles will not get the right message. We believe every disc golfer has the potential to play better, and that a strong commitment to training your mind is critical to playing your best.

You must commit to being aware of the mental frames and cognitive strategies you choose to use, and to learning to develop them to enrich your disc golf game (and perhaps your life). To help you along in this journey, we will introduce 10 essential lessons in this chapter that will lay a strong foundation for your success. We hope these lessons will not only lower your disc golf score but, more important, help you realize disc golf offers lessons that supersede mere mastery of the game.

Lesson 1: Focus on Learning and Enjoyment

There are hundreds of published books about the psychology of sports. One of our favorites is a book called *The Inner Game of Golf* by W. Timothy Gallwey. In his book, Gallwey explains what he calls the performance triangle in detail. This triangle incorporates the three central purposes associated with all human activity: learning/growth/transformation, expectations/desired results, and engaging/experiencing for pure enjoyment. As Gallwey explains, the key to realizing the three purposes lies in the way we choose to manage and operate our mind-set.

We prefer our version of a performance triangle because it illustrates the nonlinear relationship between learning, performance, and enjoyment. The three central purposes of the triangle are linked through adaptation, growth, and engagement.

You might enter into an experience because you want to learn something, acquire something

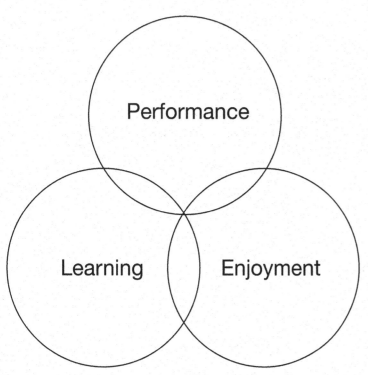

The relationship between learning, performance, and enjoyment.
Image courtesy of Justin Menickelli

tangible, or just take pleasure from experiencing something. Each of the three central purposes shapes our mind-set and influences the different activities we seek. Oftentimes, we engage in an activity and only focus on one of the three purposes, while ignoring or dismissing the others. This often-unconscious choice not only minimizes the experience, but has the potential to set us up for unnecessary drama and nonproductive distractions. This is often the case when you focus only on achieving desired results, or performance. When you only focus on results, you are unintentionally setting yourself up for disappointment, because when you do not get what you desire, it is very easy to become frustrated, angry, or depressed.

Many readers have undoubtedly experienced this phenomenon on a disc golf course. Perhaps you have a desire to earn a score below par on a particular course, and you know it is feasible because you have done it numerous times before. However, you are not playing well and you seem to be consistently hitting trees, resulting in three bogeys in the first five holes. This leads to agitation, frustration, and anger. Your choice of words to yourself and others may be negative or unbecoming, and may add fuel to the negative fire burning inside you. The reason you are frustrated has a lot to do with an attachment to your desired result. Often this frustration and negativity continues to get you further away from attaining what you desire, likely resulting in a round of disc golf you wish had never happened.

Of course, it is important to have desired outcomes and to learn to manifest what you desire in life; but it is critical not to allow your failures to spin you further away from your goals. When you intentionally choose to enter an activity with all three purposes in your mind, your thoughts begin to shift, and you do not create your own pitfalls. While playing disc golf, make a conscious choice to focus on learning and enjoyment, and not simply performance outcomes. By learning more about your game, you will begin to make adaptations and perform better. When you experience the joy of playing, you will become more engaged in the learning process and grow from the experience. Take a deep breath, pay close attention to all the wonderful, natural energy that surrounds you, engage with your fellow players, and always remember you are blessed to be playing. Presence and play are foundational components to success and happiness in every aspect of life.

Once you learn to incorporate these purposes into your game, you will find your game takes less effort and bad scoring rounds can be salvaged. More important, you will unearth a deeper meaning during the round, which can help nourish your soul long after the round is complete. Make a commitment to recognize when you are in a place of negativity fueled by your attachment to immediate results, and instead focus on learning and enjoyment of the game.

Lesson 2: Develop a Self-Referenced View of Ability and Success

There are two predominant perspectives when it comes to achievement and motivation in sport: **ego orientation** and **task orientation**. These two perspectives relate to the ways in which people perceive their level of competence. **Perceived competence** is how a person rates his or her own ability to perform well, and it can have a significant impact on effort, persistence, satisfaction, and performance.

The emphasis of an ego orientation is demonstrating superior competence. If you are an ego-oriented person, your perceived ability and success is norm-referenced. In other words, you frequently compare your attributes and outcomes to those of others. During competition, your primary objective is beating others with minimal effort, and in life and work it is being on top of everything. Reflect on your childhood and think of your annoying, adolescent neighbor beating you in a game of basketball or tennis. You may remember him or her claiming, "I beat you, and I didn't even try hard." Ego-oriented disc golfers tend to avoid improving their skills and instead simply want to compete against others they feel they can beat. When faced with adversity, these players exhibit less effort or lose interest in playing altogether. Ego-oriented players believe failure is the result of a task being too difficult for anyone to realistically accomplish, or simply bad luck.

A task orientation means perceptions of ability and success are self-referenced. When players adopt this orientation, they focus on skill improvement and being actively engaged during both practice and competitive rounds. Adopting a task-oriented, self-referenced view of ability and success leads to a strong work ethic, persistence, satisfaction, and optimal performance. When faced with adversity, task-oriented players tend to rely on using skillful performance as a way to overcome challenges. These players believe that failure is the result of a lack of skill, and that disappointment can be overcome with additional skill practice and persistence.

How do you develop a self-referenced view of ability and success? Instead of trying to be the best player among your friends or the best in your local club, make it your goal to become the best player *you can be*, through skill practice and by enjoying the experience. When you improve your skills, you gain confidence in your own ability to perform and tend to enjoy playing more than simply competing. During competitive rounds, it is not advantageous to hyper-focus on what fellow competitors are doing. Play your game, give every throw your best effort, and—again—focus on learning and enjoyment. During the last few holes of a tournament, you should be aware if you are in contention so you can strategize a bit, but strategizing is not the same as dwelling on what types of throws others are using or how well (or poorly) others are playing.

Lesson 3: Set Goals for Personal Growth

Goal setting is an excellent way to achieve personal growth and perform at your best. Setting goals can decrease your anxiety, boost your confidence, and sustain your motivation. In fact, sports psychology research indicates that goal setting can undoubtedly and consistently increase performance. In a way, committing to a systematic goal-setting program is like devoting significant time to practice putting: most people think it is a great idea, but few get around to actually doing it. Our hope is that after reading this section, you will begin to understand more about setting goals and take the time needed to effectively set them in your life.

There are several different types of goals. Subjective goals (e.g., having fun) differ from general objective goals (e.g., winning a tournament) and specific objective goals (e.g., increasing your driving distance). In addition, outcome goals (e.g., beating someone) differ from performance goals (e.g., improving your score from the previous round) and process goals (e.g., focusing on executing a proper putting stance). Setting specific objective goals that focus on both performance and process is the best strategy. Before you start working on your personal goals, we offer the following recommendations based on both relevant research and personal experience.

Set both short-range and long-range goals, and write them down. Short-range goals can help keep you motivated because you can see immediate improvements in your game. Long-range goals assist you in staying focused on what is important in your game. We recommend setting long-range goals that are not too far in the future—about a calendar year in advance is a good time frame. When you write out your goals, put one long-range goal at the top of the page. Set several progressive, short-range goals that lead up to the long-range goal, and list them below the long-range goal, with the first one that you want to accomplish at the bottom of the page. In this way, you are climbing a ladder to success. Make sure you write down target dates for each short-range and long-range goal.

Set positive—not negative—goals, and avoid setting too many goals. Three or four long-range goals related to your disc golf game are ample. Frame your goals in a positive statement. For example, "I will make 100 percent of putts shorter than 25 feet," rather than "I won't miss any short putts." Focus on success rather than failure.

Set goals for practice and competition. Getting motivated to play in a competitive environment is easy for most of us to do. Finding the motivation to practice is another story. Even if you are playing a fun, casual round with friends, it is important to set goals to help stay inspired to improve. They can be simple goals, such as, "I will approach every lie with a strategy in mind" or "I will check the wind before every drive."

Set specific goals that are measurable, attainable, and challenging. General goals such as "I want to drive well" will do little to motivate you and keep you focused. Specific, measurable goals, such as "I want the disc to land in 16 of 18 fairways," can better assist in facilitating behavior changes necessary to make them happen. Challenging yourself can be motivating, but setting unattainable goals can be deflating. For example, if you landed your disc in 8 out of 18 fairways the last time you played a course, setting a short-range goal of hitting 16 of 18 fairways may be unrealistic. Remember, progression is important.

Set both performance goals and process goals. Nearly everyone wants to win, but winning is always dependent on both factors that we can and cannot control. It is wise to judge success or failure in terms of your own performance and not on the performance of others. If you perform your best at a tournament but lose to a fellow competitor, were you not successful? Focusing only on outcome goals can be distracting, because you will concern yourself more with results than task-relevant strategies. Process goals make great short-range goals, because they assist in reminding you what you need to do to accomplish your long-range goal. Suppose your long-range goal is to throw 90 percent of your upshots within 25 feet of the target, and you are currently 60 percent accurate. What process can you improve on to reach your goal? Perhaps you can create more versatility in your game by practicing a variety of throws. This elicits a goal of practicing your forehand throw for 20 minutes each day.

Allow for goal support and evaluation. Share your goals with a coach, teacher, friend, or family member who is a good listener, a positive communicator, and is knowledgeable about setting and reaching goals. If you are new to disc golf, share your goals with someone who has years of experience playing.

Lesson 4: Focus on Aspects You Can Control

Our number one resource on the disc golf course (and in life) is how we choose to use our energy in a moment of time. You must learn to accept errant throws and take action that gets you back on track. Think about how you could have corrected the throw, and quickly move on to executing the next throw properly. This is a matter of taking responsibility and learning to focus your energy on aspects you *can* control. It has everything to do with learning to consciously choose your attitude. You should not waste your energy on aspects that you cannot control, such as changing your past shot, being in a different foursome, making the rain stop, settling down the wind, making a small tree limb disappear, erasing three bogeys you have already scored, or having more room on the tee pad.

If you really think about it, a significant percentage of what happens to you in life is out of your control. The only aspect you have control over in your life is what you choose to do in a moment of time—how you focus your energy and frame your mental perspective. Unconsciously, you may tie up your intelligence and creativity in things over which you have no control. You should make a conscious choice to free up this resistant energy and focus on acknowledgment, acceptance, and appropriate action.

You can control your reactions to any situation, including the way you react to your poorly executed throws. You can control what you choose to put in your body before, during, or after a round of disc golf. You can control and choose what you want to believe or the way you mentally frame circumstances and events. On the disc golf course, you can choose not to waste your energy dwelling on the shot that did not go your way, or complaining about the tee pads, or being distracted by other players' comments. We believe the same is true in your life and your work. You should focus all your energy on engaging in actions that create a state of flow.

Lesson 5: Create a State of Flow

A state of flow is a mental state of operation in which you are fully immersed in a feeling of energized focus, full involvement, and enjoyment. Flow is characterized by complete absorption, feelings of serenity, a loss of self-consciousness, and such a heightened focus on the present that you lose track of time passing. A flow state while playing can elicit feelings of natural joy and even ecstasy. To learn more about flow theory, we recommended a landmark book titled *Flow in Sports: The Keys to Optimal Experiences and Performances* by Susan Jackson and Mihaly Csikszentmihalyi.

In disc golf, you achieve a state of flow when you are totally engaged in the game and the majority of your throws seem effortless, controlled, and ultimately successful. Creating a state of flow has a lot to do with understanding that your perception creates reality, and each thought has the ability to create a significant shift in your life experience.

A critical aspect of creating a state of flow is to accept the current reality without judgment. When you make a mistake in throwing execution, it is good to rehearse the throw again in your mind (performed correctly), but dwelling on the outcome can disrupt flow. It is important to accept the present situation and not take things personally. Succumbing to negative thoughts or reactions from others can take you away from a state of flow. If you allow negative thoughts to fester, anger can take control. When you are playing disc golf, negativity and anger are rarely going to help create a state of flow. In fact, flow states are characterized by a lack of awareness of both emotions and physical needs.

How do you create a state of flow while playing? First, it is wise to visualize each throw before you execute it (e.g., see yourself landing the disc in a specific spot on the fairway) and even wiser to mentally rehearse all the holes before you even start the round. Simply walking around the disc golf course throwing discs rarely elicits a state of flow. Second, it is important to have a good balance between the perceived challenges and

your perceived skills. Do not allow yourself to get in an ego state by attempting throws that you are unlikely to execute correctly, given your skill level. To create flow you must have confidence in your ability to perform and choose challenging but attainable tasks. Third, playing disc golf should be intrinsically rewarding. Simply stated, just the act and art of throwing should make you feel great. If your only motives for playing are extrinsic (e.g., more social recognition or winning a prize), then it is difficult to create a flow state. Last, you should believe you have personal influence over each outcome you experience. Accept both positive and negative outcomes to your performance, and do not blame the negatives on good or bad luck or other variables, like noise on the course or how strong the wind is blowing. Instead, challenge yourself to eliminate both positive and negative thinking and accept the things you cannot control.

Lesson 6: Approach Your Lie with a Preplanned Strategy

It is imperative to think about your upcoming shot before standing behind your marker disc. Once you have executed a shot and your disc has come to rest, instead of focusing on your last throw, attend to your next throw. As you are walking to the placement of your next shot, you will find you have ample time to get prepared. Use this time while approaching your lie to focus your mental energy and thought on how you plan to execute the next throw. This includes analyzing all the different variables that are in play. Where is the greatest **percentage of open space** for the next shot? Where is the optimal landing area or specific target? In what direction is the wind blowing? What type of throw is likely to give you the best results? Make a definitive decision on which throw you are going to use, then begin to focus on what the disc will look like when flying through the air. Remember to visualize both the flight and landing.

You might think it is not feasible to prepare before you actually stand behind your marker because the angles of your disc's flight pattern change once you are actually in position to throw, and you see some of the fairway variables differently. It is true that the angles will change as you approach your marker; but in many cases you can position yourself 30 to 60 feet behind your marker without bothering the other players in the group and you can begin to get a pretty accurate assessment of the upcoming throw, and best landing zone. It is important to approach your lie with thoughtfulness, because once you put your foot behind your marker, you have 30 seconds to execute your throw. Indecision and rushed throws without proper preparation often lead to poor execution. Remember to fully commit to your throw; debating in your mind during execution rarely, if ever, leads to optimal results.

Lesson 7: Focus on the Target

There is a great deal of research on the advantages of focusing externally on movement effect (e.g., the flight of the disc) verses focusing internally on movement execution (e.g., your throwing motion). Basically, when your attention is directed to the desired movement effect, you perform better than when you focus on movement execution. Also, there is evidence to suggest that focusing on movement effect improves retention of the knowledge needed to learn the skill. During

practice, especially if you are an absolute beginner, it may be a good idea to occasionally focus on your movements, such as extending your arm when you putt or tweaking your drive form to effectively load your hips. When competing, you should focus on disc flight and the optimal target and landing zone. Imagine successful outcomes, and focus very little on movement execution.

In disc golf, focusing on the target means that before you execute any throw, you want to first specifically identify the landing zone where you want your disc to come to rest. Sometimes that landing zone is the actual target, but in many cases it is on the line of trajectory you want the disc to fly. It could be a tree or other obstacle in the distance; however, it is on the exact line needed to set you up for your next shot. For throws with no sight line to the target (called blind throws), a great strategy is to aim for a tree you have no chance of hitting but one that affords the best route to the target or landing zone.

Lesson 8: Imagine Success

"Imagine it, and it can happen" might be words you find etched on a wooden plaque in a tacky gift shop, but there is strong scientific evidence that such a strategy actually works. Often used in sports contexts, **imagery** is the use of the senses to create or recreate experiences in the mind. Imagery is synonymous with terms like *visualization* and *mental practice*. We prefer the term *imagery* because it implies a polysensory experience. After all, great throws have a look, feel, and sound to them. When used immediately prior to performance execution, this strategy is called preparatory imagery. Using preparatory imagery during a round of disc golf

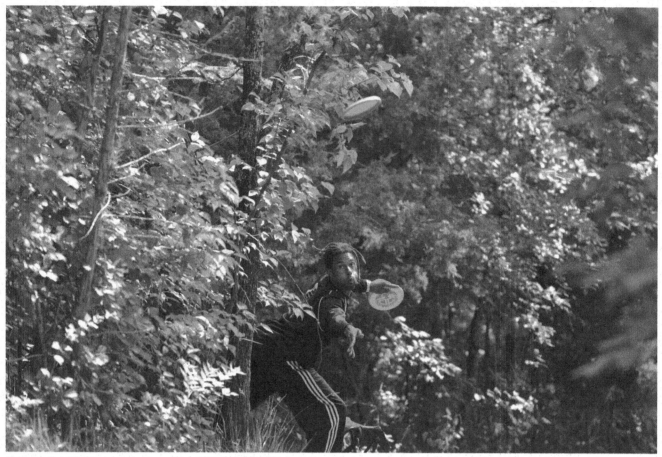

Philo Brathwaite demonstrates some creativity and versatility to get out of a jam. *Photo courtesy of PDGA Media*

can help you control your emotions, optimize your arousal level, and not only facilitate how you perform but how you respond to the stress of competition.

How does it work? Well, there are a few theories that attempt to explain how imagery works, but there is little concrete evidence to exclusively support or dispute a single theory. Many people believe that it aids in achieving optimal arousal levels by helping you feel relaxed but stimulated enough to focus your attention on what is important.

Certain sports and skills are more conducive to using preparatory imagery than others. Preparatory

imagery is most effective when executing closed skills such as hitting a golf ball, kicking a field goal, shooting free throws, and throwing a disc. Using preparatory imagery for open skills like surfing in the ocean, avoiding defenders in soccer, or executing a fast break in basketball is not as effective. Jack Nicklaus (arguably the best traditional golfer of all time) and Dick Fosbury (the 1968 Olympic gold medalist in the high jump and inventor of the revolutionary Fosbury Flop) were just two of many successful athletes who used preparatory imagery. Both Nicklaus and Fosbury often appeared laser-focused before execution, seemingly muttering to themselves. At first, their approach caused many to laugh; nobody is laughing now. Utilizing a relatively simple preparatory imagery strategy can help make you a better disc golfer.

As you approach your marker, imagine what different throws will look, feel, and sound like. Next, as discussed earlier, make a definitive decision on which throw you will execute. Then take a few seconds to imagine what your specific throw will look, feel, and sound like. Grip the disc and allow the tactile sensation to flow from your fingertips, and take a few deep breaths. Engage in some positive self-talk by telling yourself what will happen and visualizing the throw. Focus on the flight of the disc, from release to landing. Imagine success and not failure. Avoid imagining hitting the first tree on the fairway or your disc landing in the pond. While putting, imagine the disc entering the target and hear the sounds of the rattling chains.

Beginners can use imagery techniques to get a mental blueprint of the skill and as a way to stay motivated to improve. Experts use it to build confidence, to deeply ingrain the perfect mental blueprint, and to develop strategy. Regardless of your skill level or experience, imagery takes practice. You should use this relatively simple but tremendously effective technique during both practice and competitive rounds as often as possible. Do not get frustrated if you do not see results immediately.

Before a competitive round, use imagery in the form of mental practice. Take the time to walk the course so you can blueprint the fairways and target placements in your mind. Review each hole in your mind and imagine what executing a successful drive looks, feels, and sounds like. Imagine executing effective upshots and successful putts. Allow these images to permeate your body. Some players find it is easier to write down a script that specifies everything they want to remember. In doing so, you can review the script and create the movie in your mind.

Lesson 9: Build Confidence with Self-Talk

It is important to understand that our thoughts directly impact our feelings and ultimately our behaviors. Confident players think about themselves, and the task at hand, in a different way than those who lack confidence. Confidence is a result of particular thinking habits more so than raw talent or previous success. When practiced intentionally and consistently, these thinking habits can become natural and automatic. Players can retain and benefit from successful experiences and restructure memories or feelings from less successful experiences. In essence, both successes and failures can allow you to build confidence. One can choose to believe there is no such thing as failures, only opportunities to learn and grow.

You engage in self-talk any time you have a dialogue with yourself. This can be instructional (e.g., "Pop your wrist") or motivational (e.g., "Nice recovery throw"). This dialogue may occur out loud for extroverts and internally, in silence, for introverts. Self-talk is advantageous when it enhances overall self-worth and performance, as it can help you stay focused on immediate success. It can also assist in not dwelling on mistakes, such as a missed putt, and not focusing on the future (for example, obsessing over needing a birdie to get to even par for the round).

Negative self-talk, such as "I suck at putting," is detrimental and should be avoided. If you train your mind to engage in an adequate amount of positive self-talk, you can reduce thought patterns that lead to errors and permit automatic execution of the skills needed to play well. It is appropriate for self-talk during practice to focus on mechanics (extending your arm, for example). During competitive rounds, self-talk should focus on desired feelings (e.g., smooth and easy) or a desired outcome (e.g., center chains). Avoid talking about what not to do ("Don't hit that tree"); keep your self-talk statements positive and brief.

Talking to yourself may seem silly, but it can improve your attentional focus, allow you to change a bad habit, and help maintain energy and persistence. With practice, positive self-talk regimens can build confidence and facilitate learning and performance. Awareness is the first step to all transformation, and requires people to witness their own presence as if they were a director overseeing the making of a movie. Once you are conscious of your thinking, your feelings and ultimately your behaviors can be modified through intentional choice. Engaging in effective self-talk regimens takes practice, but committing to improving self-talk can be a rewarding experience.

Lesson 10: Develop Versatility and Creativity in Your Game

The ability to be versatile and creative is critical in many sports. In disc golf, versatility is the ability to execute many types of throws, and creativity is having the experience to recognize when to use them. Versatility allows us to take different paths or courses of action, and when aligned with the path of the least resistance, can help elicit success. Being creative does not mean taking great risks, because

the path of least resistance is often the best choice. Similar to a river or creek, water always flows along the path of the least resistance. It finds the cracks, the gullies, and the small holes to flow through. From this lesson in nature, we can learn to identify the path of least resistance. In disc golf, this path is often the greatest percentage of open space.

The difference between playing well and scoring well often comes down to versatility. Executing various throwing styles (e.g., forehand, backhand, **roller**, **thumber**, etc.) allows a player to take advantage of the greatest percentage of open space. Of course, developing different throwing styles takes physical practice, but developing the ability to recognize when to use them takes mental practice and experience. Once you are able to achieve versatility and creativity in your game, you will have better options to approach any target and will become an excellent scrambler. You will have the ability to get out of difficult situations (i.e., poor lies) by identifying the best path and performing various types of throws.

Cultivating versatility and creativity takes practice and experience, but there are ways to encourage their development during a round. Indeed, it can be advantageous to create versatility during a competitive round when you are having difficulty creating a state of flow. This can be accomplished by self-selecting different throwing techniques, or using a disc you would not normally use for a given throw. For example, you could choose to throw a backhand **anhyzer** in lieu of a forehand **hyzer** to navigate a similar route (more on throwing styles later). You could choose to putt with a midrange disc or drive with a putter. In doing this, you can trigger a mental switch that permits you to think differently about a round.

Chapter 6

Disc Golf Fitness

n this chapter, we prescribe a fitness regimen that includes a dynamic warm-up, a cooldown, **flexibility** training, and functional strength training. The recommended progressive warm-up routine will make you physically and mentally ready to play, and it functions as quality skill practice. Following the recommendations outlined in this chapter may help a player of any age avoid painful damage to muscles and joints. In essence, if you adhere to this fitness routine, you will find that you will not only play better, but feel better.

Disc golf is a sport that requires players to demonstrate explosive power and functional flexibility. These attributes can be improved by simply playing disc golf, but if you follow the suggestions presented in this book, you can develop them more rapidly while avoiding injuries. Unlike the more aerobically strenuous game of Ultimate, there is no evidence to suggest that being in phenomenal aerobic shape will make you a better disc golfer. Nevertheless, if you are in poor enough aerobic shape that you often stand over putts with your heart pounding after walking up a gentle hill, some aerobic conditioning can improve your game tremendously.

Similar to playing traditional golf, disc golf is predominantly an asymmetrical activity. In other words, players typically throw using their preferred arm, which asymmetrically applies stress on their dominant shoulder, elbow, and knee joint. As such, skeletomuscular and articular injuries are common. Playing disc golf necessitates unilateral rotation of the hip, and thus injuries to the lower spine are also fairly common. Using different throwing styles may help combat this tendency, but physical conditioning is the best way to ensure you develop the symmetrical muscular strength and joint flexibility needed to play your best while avoiding injury. If you play disc golf just for fun, remember that playing well and staying injury-free is always fun.

Warming Up

Warming up is a critical part of performing well in any sport. If you do not devote the time to properly warm up before playing, you may not perform at your best and you may increase the likelihood of getting injured. Many disc golfers simply show up to the course, throw a few drives from the first tee pad, and then start playing. However, the best way to be both physically and mentally ready to play well is to warm up properly. Developing a consistent warm-up routine has many specific physiological benefits, including raising the heart rate, increasing body and tissue temperature, increasing blood flow to active muscles, increasing the speed at which nerve impulses travel, increasing synovial fluid production, improving joint quality, increasing muscular efficiency, and decreasing muscular tension.

These physiological variables are closely related to the psychological benefits of warming up. When you step on the first tee pad to start a round, it is natural for your body to show signs of anxiety and a spike in arousal level. Heart rate, blood pressure, breathing rate, sweating, muscle tension, and even brain wave activity can all increase substantially under the psychological pressure of trying to perform a great throw. These physiological responses can wreak havoc on attentional focus and the ability to perform well. By properly warming up, these physiological responses increase gradually, allowing you to better focus on successful outcomes. In essence, warming up physically and mentally go hand in hand.

Developing a consistent warm-up routine will make you a better disc golfer, because in addition to getting your body physically and mentally ready, it can also function as quality skill-specific practice. To take advantage of this motor skill learning benefit, we recommend devoting at least one hour to warming up before every disc golf outing. In colder weather, warming up properly will take longer. The preponderance of published research indicates that **stretching** before warming up is not only ineffective, but potentially harmful. In fact, static stretching before physical performance can

have a negative impact on **force** production. As a result, we do not recommend stretching before a round. Instead, we recommend a dynamic and progressive warm-up routine, followed by static stretching during the cooldown period.

Suggested Warm-Up Routine

Stage 1 (10 minutes): Walk for about 10 minutes at low to moderate intensity (a comfortable but fairly brisk pace). If you are lucky enough to live close to your favorite course, walking or riding a bike to the course is a great way to begin your routine. Walking the first six holes of the course is a good strategy as well. Use this time to hydrate before you feel thirsty. This initial bout of exercise will slowly elevate your heart rate, breathing rate, core temperature, and blood flow to your muscles, and as a result, you should start to sweat.

Stage 2 (10 minutes): Avoid the crowded putting target and find a hole not in use. Grab five putters and start warming up your mind and body for putting. Start about 20 feet from the target and putt five times in succession. Take a step after each put in either a clockwise or counterclockwise direction to allow for different wind direction. Gradually increase your distance to the target and putt using both a traditional and **straddle stance** (more on stances later). Attempt a variety of putts (e.g., uphill, downhill, from behind a tree, etc.). Before each attempt, imagine the disc hitting the chains. After you let the disc go, focus on the flight of the disc and where it hits the chains. When you miss a putt, perform a quick self-evaluation and make corrections. For example, adjust your aim or set your feet correctly. Focus chiefly on being successful but do not fret over missed putts. Feel good about the fact that you are now getting properly warmed up and ready to play your best.

Stage 3 (10 minutes): Find a partner who shares your passion for the game and a soft, blunt-edge putter. Do not use a midrange disc or driver. Begin by standing about 50 feet apart and smoothly throw the putter back and forth. Throw using a variety of styles (backhand, **forehand**, etc.) at various **throwing angles** (hyzer and anhyzer). Perform five throws of the same style before switching. After about five minutes, gradually increase the distance between you and your partner to between 80 and 100 feet and continue throwing for another five minutes. Occasionally shift your attentional focus inward to monitor your throwing intensity. Remember, the idea is to gradually increase the intensity of your throws.

Of course, you do not need to practice catching (like you would for a game of Ultimate), but this is an efficient way to warm up, and you only need one disc. If you cannot find a partner or you choose not to use one, find an open area or a fairway not in use, grab your five favorite putters, and utilize the same basic procedure (minus the catches, of course). If you choose a fairway on the course, do not worry about **holing out** on each throw; simply focus on the flight of the disc and hitting the target or landing area. This routine will gradually and specifically warm up your body for throwing.

Stage 4 (15 minutes): Find a hole on the course not in use and select your five favorite midrange discs. Position yourself about 100 feet from the target or selected landing area and throw each midrange disc using one throwing style. Repeat this step using other throwing styles. Gradually increase the intensity of your throws as you slowly increase your distance from the target. If you need a driver to reach the target, then you are too far away. Before each throw, imagine the flight you want the disc to take and where you want it to land. This

stage of the warm-up routine continues to warm up your body for throwing. As discussed in the previous chapter, it will also help you optimize your attentional focus by practicing preparatory imagery. It may sound silly, but imagining success really does help facilitate desired performance.

Stage 5 (15 minutes): Find a tee pad not in use and practice your driving approach steps without a disc. Imagine the flight of a perfectly thrown disc, and it landing in an ideal spot on the fairway or green. At this stage, you should be properly warmed up enough to load your hips (wind your spine) and throw drives with explosive power. Throw three to six drives using a midrange, fairway driver, or driver disc, and do not forget to imagine the ideal flight before each throw. Retrieve your discs, and then go to the next hole you want to practice. Throw each driver again and focus on successful outcomes. Putt out some or all of the drives during this stage, but do not fret over missed putts.

If you are playing in a tournament, warming up properly can be problematic, because after you have warmed up, you may be asked to sit for 15 to 60 minutes. The general protocol is for tournament directors to hold a mandatory players' meeting immediately before all the players are sent out to their first hole in a shotgun-start format. During these meetings, TDs review important information about the course and rules of play. They often bring attention to sponsors and volunteers that have helped make the tournament possible. Although necessary, these meetings typically occur at the worst possible time—immediately after players have warmed up. Players' meetings that occur the evening before a tournament, or even a few hours before, provide more warm-up-friendly options. We do not recommend missing players' meetings,

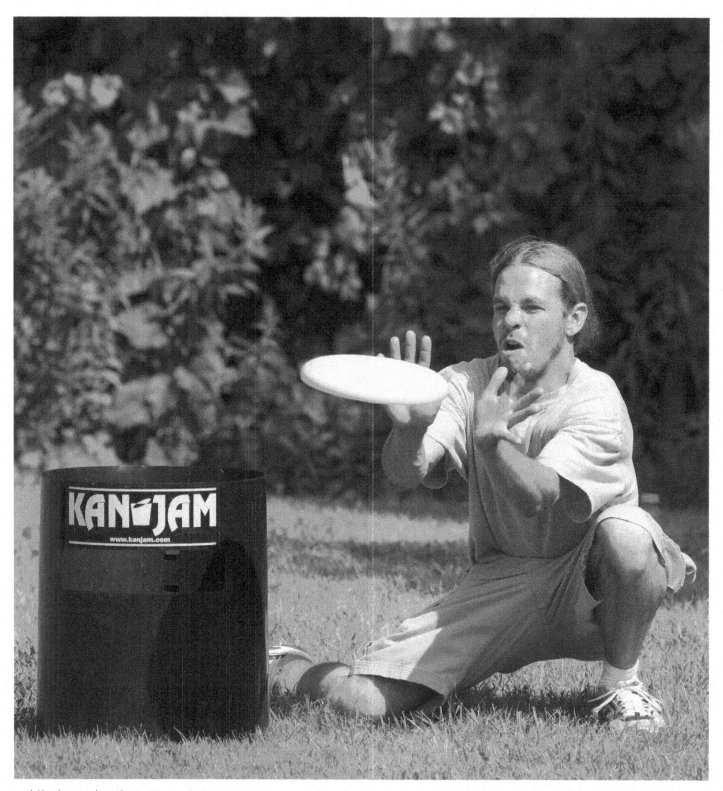

A KanJammer in action. *Photo courtesy of kanjam.com*

although we understand doing so may help avoid the dreaded cooldown effect.

If you want to try a different, exciting warm-up routine, consider playing a game of **KanJam**. It is essentially a more physically active version of horseshoes or cornhole, played with a disc. You will need four people, one throw-and-catch type of disc, and two cylindrical KanJam goals. If you have been to a disc golf or Ultimate tournament, then you have probably seen folks playing this game in the evenings, following competition. Of course, the game does not provide all the elements of the recommended warm-up routine, but it may be too much fun to resist playing as an alternative once in a while.

Cooling Down

A proper cooldown after a round of disc golf is almost as important as warming up. It is imperative to provide your body time to adjust from a period of exercise to rest. Although many disc golfers prefer to sit in a chair and enjoy a cold beverage, we recommend beginning your cooldown routine by walking at low intensity for about 10 minutes. In this way, you can reduce the pooling of metabolic waste and gradually calm your neuromuscular system to enter a period of relaxation and regeneration. If possible, carry only water and rehydrate frequently. This is the best time to incorporate flexibility training, because tissue temperatures will be highest during this period.

Flexibility Training

Flexibility is the capability to move muscles and joints through their full range of motion. Stretching is the process of elongating muscles and connective tissues. The suggested warm-up routine presented in this book will assist in developing functional flexibility. Stretching during the cooldown period can significantly reduce the risk of joint sprain and muscle strain, while also reducing muscle soreness and tension.

The approach we recommend for improving flexibility during the cooldown period involves static stretching. This method is the safest and easiest to learn, and it requires little energy expenditure. Static stretching can improve flexibility but does very little (if anything) to improve coordination and muscular force production and, as a result, it does not replace a progressive, dynamic warm-up routine. Again, we strongly recommend performing static stretching exercises after but not before playing disc golf.

The bad news is that flexibility tends to decrease with age, but the good news is that it can be developed at any age. You may find that performing the classic yoga poses and stretches we recommend in sequence provides tremendous benefits. We recommend them because they stretch the major muscles used for playing disc golf, and they do not require equipment or a partner. Of course, there are other stretching techniques that may be of personal benefit.

We recommend performing your stretches without distraction so you can focus your attention internally on taking deep, controlled breaths and relaxing certain muscles while activating others. Perform two to five repetitions for each stretch, holding each for about 15 to 20 seconds. If your muscles start to quiver, you experience painful surges, or your range of motion decreases, you have stretched too much and should cease performing the stretches immediately.

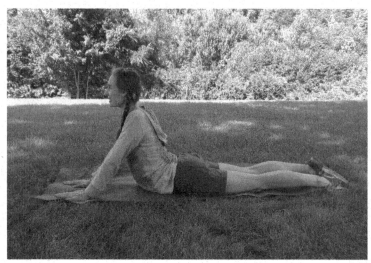

Upward facing dog. *Photo courtesy of Justin Menickelli*

Upward Facing Dog

- A classic yoga pose that stretches abdominal muscles
- Lie flat on the ground with palms facedown by the middle of your ribs
- Draw your legs together and press the tops of your feet into the ground using your back, not hands, to gently lift your chest off the ground
- Note: Leave legs extended straight out and take deep, controlled breaths

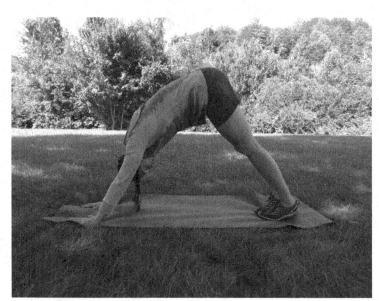

Downward facing dog. *Photo courtesy of Justin Menickelli*

Downward Facing Dog

- A classic yoga pose that stretches gluteus (maximus, medius, and minimus muscles), hamstrings, gastrocnemius, and deltoids
- Start on all fours with hands directly under shoulders and knees under hips
- Walk hands a few inches forward and spread fingers wide, pressing palms into ground
- Curl toes under and slowly press hips upward, bringing your body into an inverted *V* by pressing shoulders away from ears
- Feet should be hip width apart, knees slightly bent
- Note: press through the arms and fingers and take deep, controlled breaths

Modified Hurdler's Stretch

- Stretches hamstrings
- Sit on the ground with one leg straight and the other bent at the knee
- Place heel touching inside of thigh
- Lower outside of thigh and calf of bent leg to the ground
- Keep extended leg straight and lower upper torso while exhaling slowly
- Switch legs and repeat
- Note: focus on contracting your quadriceps to relax your hamstrings

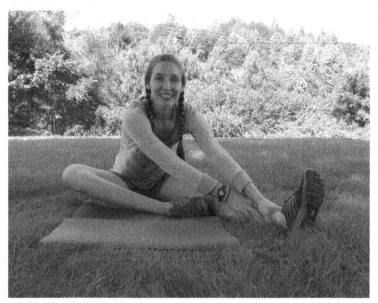

Modified hurdler's stretch. *Photo courtesy of Justin Menickelli*

Butterfly Stretch

- Stretches adductor muscles of the upper thigh
- Sit on the ground with hips flexed and spread, and heels touching
- Grasp feet or ankles and pull them close to groin
- Place elbows on inner thighs and knees, exhale, and push legs toward the ground
- Note: be sure your back is straight when performing this stretch

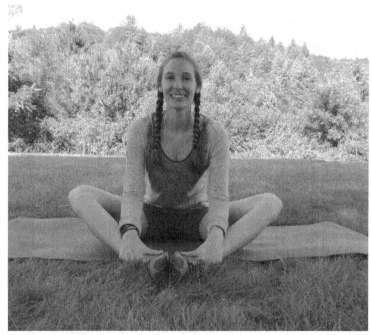

Butterfly stretch. *Photo courtesy of Justin Menickelli*

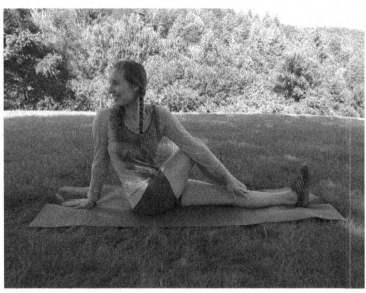

Seated spiral stretch. *Photo courtesy of Justin Menickelli*

Seated Spiral Stretch

- Stretches the gluteus muscles of the hip and buttocks
- Sit on the ground with hands behind hips and legs extended
- Cross left foot over right leg and slide heel toward buttocks
- Place right elbow outside left knee
- Exhale and look over left shoulder while turning trunk and gently pushing on knee with right elbow
- Switch legs and repeat

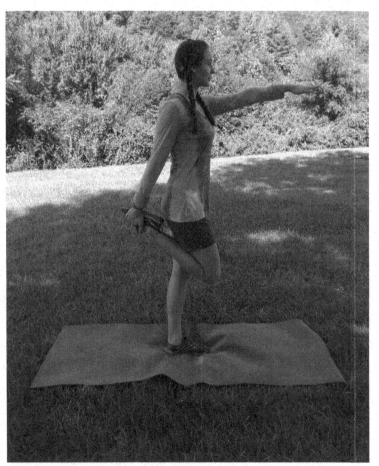

Standing quad stretch. *Photo courtesy of Justin Menickelli*

Standing Quad Stretch

- Stretches quadriceps muscles of the legs
- Stand holding onto something for balance, if possible
- Flex one knee and raise heel to buttocks
- Slightly flex supporting leg, exhale, and grasp raised foot
- Inhale and slowly pull heel toward buttocks
- Inside of legs should be touching and pelvis should rotate backward
- Switch legs and repeat
- Note: do not arch your lower back or twist pelvis

Lateral Shoulder Stretch

- Stretches the deltoids and infraspinatus muscles of the shoulder
- Stand with one arm raised to shoulder height
- Flex arm across other shoulder
- Grasp raised elbow with opposite hand, exhale, and pull elbow backward
- Switch arms and repeat

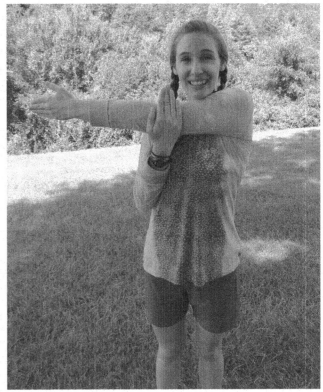

Lateral shoulder stretch. *Photo courtesy of Justin Menickelli*

Back Scratch Stretch

- Stretches the triceps muscle of the arm
- Stand with one arm flexed, raised overhead next to ear, and hand on shoulder blade
- Grasp elbow with other hand, exhale, and pull elbow behind head

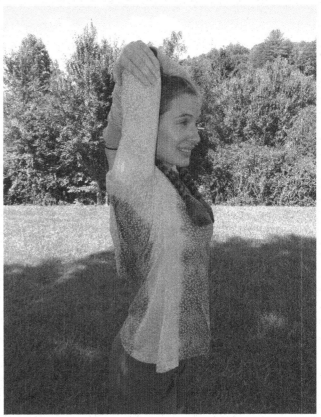

Back scratch stretch. *Photo courtesy of Justin Menickelli*

Functional Strength Training

You do not have to lift weights to improve muscular strength and endurance to a degree that will enhance your disc golf game. Many professional players devote time to lifting weights during the off-season, but simply performing the following six exercises may do a lot to improve your game. Performing these exercises two to three times a week can assist in developing the arm, leg, back, abdominal, and hip muscles used when playing disc golf. The emphasis is on developing the core muscles of your abdominals, back, and hips needed to throw discs with power.

Concentrating on functional strength training can help you avoid injury, aid in developing symmetrical musculature, and assist in improving explosive power and balance. We should note here that maximal strength gains are obtained when you perform any exercise to the point of muscular failure (the point at which you cannot perform more repetitions due to fatigue). We do not recommend performing the suggested exercises to failure to prevent straining a muscle, but doing them until you are considerably fatigued will result in significant strength gains. Each of the exercises is designed to strengthen your core muscles. Your core is composed of many different muscles in your abdomen, back, sides, pelvis, and buttocks that work together to allow you to bend, twist, and rotate. We recommend acquiring three medicine balls that weigh about two, three, and five kilograms to assist in developing core strength.

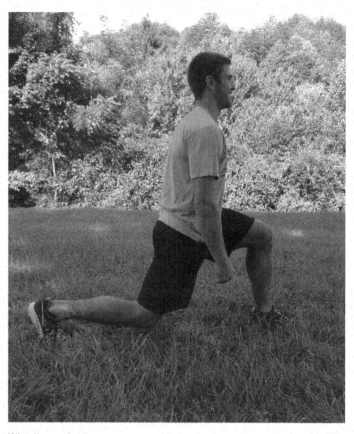

Wheelhouse lunge. *Photo courtesy of Justin Menickelli*

Wheelhouse Lunges

- Stand with feet about hip width apart and slightly bend knees
- Contract abdominal muscles and relax shoulders
- Take big steps forward, backward, sideways, and diagonal, and alternate your lead leg
- Keep your back as straight as possible
- Note: your knee should never go past the outstretched foot

Back-to-Back Rotations

- Stand back-to-back with partner of about same height
- Smoothly pass medicine ball to each other by rotating hips
- Keep ball just above waist height
- Perform for three to five minutes, then pass ball in other direction
- Note: the ball should feel heavy but comfortable in your arms

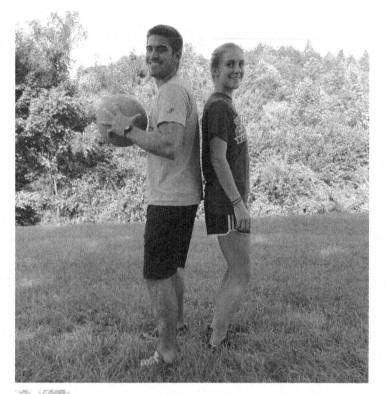

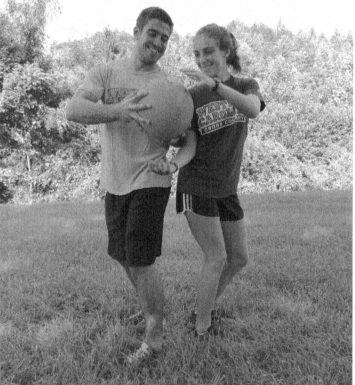

Back-to-back rotation. *Photos courtesy of Justin Menickelli*

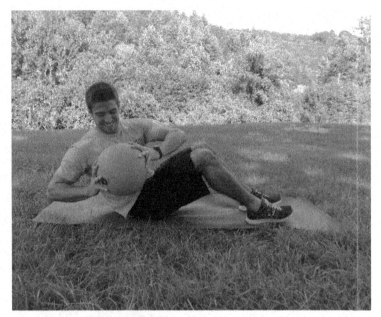

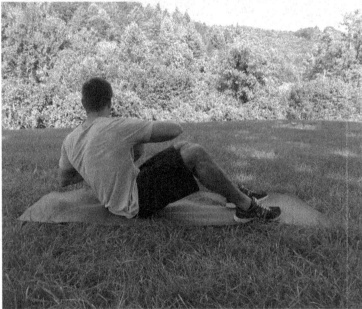

Back-to-back rotation. *Photos courtesy of Justin Menickelli*

Torso Rotations

- Sit on the ground with knees bent, feet flat on the ground, holding ball at chest with both hands
- Lean torso away from thighs, increasing angle at hips and contracting abdominals
- Maintain hip angle, smoothly rotate torso to the right, moving right elbow toward the ground behind you
- Return to center position and smoothly rotate to the left
- Repeat 10 to 20 times for each side

Reverse Crunches

- Lie on ground on your back, with knees bent and hands behind head
- Lift legs and bend knees to 90°
- Keep a space between your chin and chest, looking at the sky
- Exhale and pull your knees toward your chest
- Inhale and slowly lower legs back to starting position
- Note: do not use your momentum to swing your legs up. Try to keep the motion controlled by your lower abdominal muscles.

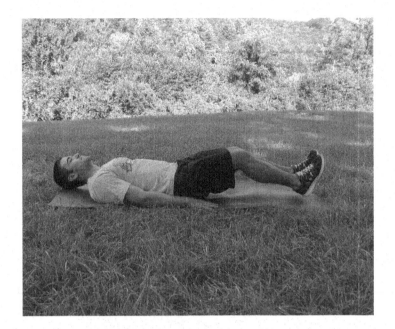

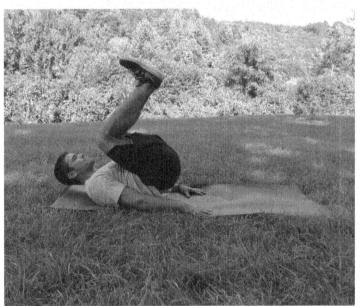

Reverse crunch. *Photos courtesy of Justin Menickelli*

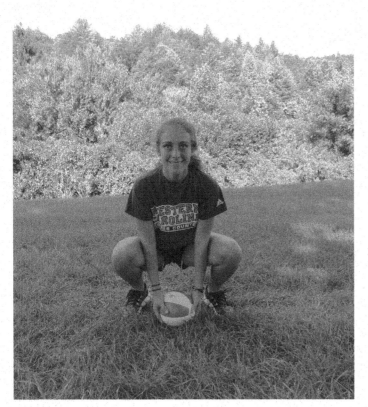

Squats with Overhead Lift

- Stand with feet wider than shoulder width, holding ball with both hands
- Flex knees while lowering buttocks and knees over ankles
- Keep back straight and head neutral
- Return to starting position and quickly but smoothly lift medicine ball overhead
- Repeat squat and lower ball to ground for 10 to 20 repetitions
- Note: Olympic shot-putters perform a similar exercise that entails explosively tossing the shot put backward over their heads. Safety is obviously paramount if you choose to perform this technique.

Squat with overhead lift. *Photos courtesy of Justin Menickelli*

Push-ups with Hip Extensions

- On hands and knees, place hands about shoulder width apart
- Extend right leg straight back and contract abdominal muscles
- Keep leg lifted and lower chest to ground until elbows are at 90° angle, then push upward
- Repeat 10 to 20 times with each leg
- Note: keep your head neutral while performing this exercise

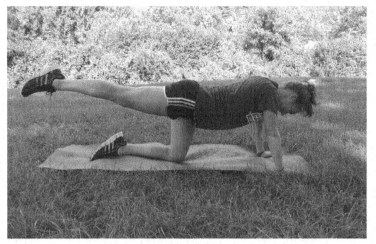

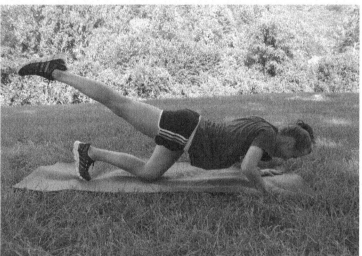

Push-ups with hip extensions. *Photos courtesy of Justin Menickelli*

Aerobic Training

Regardless of your age, aerobic training is beneficial for all. As your body adapts to regular aerobic exercise, you will undoubtedly become stronger and you will feel more fit. You may also feel less tension associated with anxiety and be more relaxed. During aerobic activity, you raise your metabolic rate, which leads to increased ventilation in response to an increase in oxygen kinetics. Your heart rate increases to help supply blood flow to your active muscles and back to your lungs. Your skeletal muscle capillaries dilate to enhance oxygen delivery to your muscles and improve metabolic waste removal. As your heart gets stronger, it does not need to beat as fast at rest, and it pumps blood more efficiently.

Of course, playing disc golf does not require you to run, but running for at least 20 minutes three or more times a week can improve your game, especially during the last round of a four-or-more-round tournament. If running does not appeal to you, a fun way to improve your aerobic conditioning is to play **speed golf**. Basically, speed golf is played with only two discs, and instead of trying to get the best possible score, the goal is to complete the course in the shortest amount of time. Some people prefer to keep score, but you do not have to. You could play with just a midrange disc and putter or try out a new disc. Basically, you start your stopwatch the moment you throw your first drive and stop it as soon as you hole out on the last hole. We typically play a round of speed golf in about 40 minutes or less through a combination of jogging and fast walking. If you regularly play rounds of speed golf, when you play a regular round it may feel like a leisurely walk in the park.

When playing speed golf, we encourage you to play during times when there are not a lot of other people on the course. As such, speed golf rounds are ideally played early in the morning or right before dusk. Playing at these times will ensure you can get out on the course and run through all the holes without having to stop to wait on others who are playing. If you encounter other players, politely hollering "Speed round!" will let people know you are playing for fitness. We find that most people let us play through, and we even get shouts of encouragement on occasion.

Chapter 7

The Dynamics of Disc Flight

This chapter addresses two fundamental but complex questions about the aerodynamics and gyrodynamics of disc flight: What effects do **velocity**, throwing angle, **drag**, **lift**, and **spin** have on the flight of a disc? Why do some discs fly differently than others? Later in this chapter, we will answer commonly asked questions about **speed**, glide, stability, and angles as they relate to golf disc selection and throwing execution. We will address the basic principles of a flying disc thrown using either a backhand or forehand (also called **sidearm**) style. Some, but not all, of the principles here apply to discs thrown using overhead (thumber or **tomahawk**) throwing styles. The impact of dynamic forces on overhead throwing styles has not yet been investigated.

Much of the research on the aerodynamic and gyrodynamic properties of flying discs has been conducted using mathematical models and wind tunnel tests. The bulk of the available data may be appealing to students studying applied aerodynamics, sport biomechanics, or astrophysics, but to the average disc golfer, it can be overwhelming. For a deep look into the dynamics of spinning flight, we recommend a fantastic book

written by Ralph Lorenz titled *Spinning Flight: Dynamics of Frisbees, Boomerangs, Samaras, and Skipping Stones*. Lorenz, an aerospace engineer–turned–planetary scientist, summarizes hundreds of studies (including his own free-flight research) on flying and spinning objects.

Golf Disc Geometry

Golf discs are composed of a rim and a center section (often referred to as the **flight plate**). Golf discs differ from throw-and-catch models (such as a Discraft Ultra-Star or Innova Pulsar) in their overall diameter, inside rim diameter, thickness, camber, rim width, and rim depth. Primarily the rim width, depth, and camber differentiate golf discs from the throw-and-catch variety. As you read in chapter 1, it was changes to the rim of a traditional Frisbee that made throwing farther possible. See the illustration of typical golf disc geometry on page 90.

A flying disc is both an airfoil (like an airplane wing) and a gyroscope (like a spinning top). Understanding disc flight begins with knowing how the two systems interact, and to the layperson, it can be a challenge to comprehend. We will begin

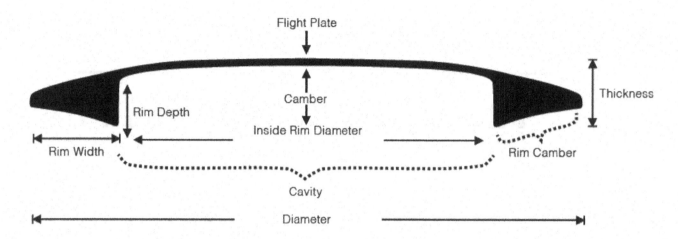

Schematic view of typical golf disc geometry. *Based on an original figure by Noorfazreena Kamaruddin*

by concisely defining some terminology that we will use throughout this chapter.

Forces, Vectors, and Moments

A force is any influence that causes an object to start, stop, speed up, slow down, or change direction. A force has both magnitude and direction, making it a **vector** quantity. A vector is a mathematical representation of anything (including forces) described by both its magnitude and direction. Vectors are often graphically represented by an arrow. **Torque** (also called **rotary force**) is the turning effect produced by a force. The **moment** of a force is a measure of its tendency to cause an object to rotate about a specific point or axis.

The forces discussed in this chapter include **gravity**, drag, lift, and **acceleration**. Gravity is a constant vertical force defined as the weight of an object. Drag acts in opposition to the relative motion of an object, whereas lift acts perpendicular to the relative motion of an object. Acceleration is

the rate of change in velocity. Since velocity is often misunderstood, we will define it in detail first.

Velocity

Most people use the terms *velocity* and *speed* interchangeably, but they are mechanically different. Speed is simply the rate of motion. Velocity indicates both magnitude and orientation (direction) and is represented by a vector (essentially an arrow that indicates direction). As a disc flies, both the magnitude and orientation are constantly changing. After all, as a disc slows down it also rises and falls. Instantaneous velocity is the velocity of an object at an instant in time. Relative velocity, in the case of flying discs, is the difference between the disc's velocity and the air velocity. Relative velocity is the magnitude of the effect of the air molecules on the disc and is important to mention before talking about aerodynamic (the motion of air) and gyrodynamic (the effect of spin) parameters. Given the same instantaneous velocity when a disc leaves your hand, a disc thrown into a headwind will have a greater relative velocity than one thrown into a tailwind. For a disc golfer, this means that a disc can be thrown farther with a slight headwind because the positive effect of greater lift typically outweighs the negative effect of additional drag forces.

Aerodynamic Forces

The two main aerodynamic forces that act on a flying disc are drag and lift. In essence, flying discs behave much like an airplane wing does. As a disc flies, air molecules exert pressure on it. This pressure, called the **dynamic fluid force**, is proportional to the air density, the surface area of the disc, and the square of the relative velocity of the disc to the air. So, if the relative velocity doubles, the dynamic fluid force roughly quadruples.

Drag forces act in opposition to the relative motion of a disc with respect to the air and tend to decrease relative velocity. Drag forces are produced by two different means: **form drag** and **surface drag**. Form drag (also called profile or shape drag) is the sum of the impact forces resulting from the collision between the air molecules and a flying disc. Form drag is most influenced by the curvature or cross-sectional area of a disc. Imagine air rushing by the top and bottom of a flying disc. As air molecules strike the surface of the disc, they bounce off, but then the air molecules strike other air molecules and are pushed back toward the surface of the disc. Air molecules on the leading edge of the disc are directed toward the trailing edge. On the trailing edge, air molecules are also directed toward the front of a disc. If the air molecules stay close to the surface, a layer of laminar (streamline or undisrupted) flow forms. However, if the impact forces between air

molecules are not large enough to deflect molecules back toward a disc's surface, the molecules separate from the surface, and thus **turbulent flow** is created. Laminar flow is linear and orderly while turbulent flow is highly irregular. The difference between the forward- and backward-directed forces is the form drag. In general, as turbulent flow increases, so does form drag.

Streamlined or gently curved shapes have less form drag than non-streamlined ones. After all, sports cars have much less form drag than minivans. In much the same way, golf discs designed for greater distance or range have more streamlined rim profiles than discs designed for shorter flights. Deep rims on the underside of discs designed for short-range throws tend to create a larger area of turbulent flow projected into the laminar flow, and thus greater drag. Subtle differences in rim width, rim depth, lower surface rim camber, or overall thickness can also have profound effects on profile drag. For example, a golf disc with a slightly wider rim (a few millimeters) can result in less form drag and thus different flight characteristics.

Surface drag (also called viscous drag), is the sum of the friction forces acting between the air molecules and the surface of a disc or the friction forces between the air molecules themselves. Rough surfaces tend to create larger friction forces between an object and air molecules. A roughed-up or worn disc (often called a seasoned disc) has greater surface drag and therefore tends to fly differently than a newer version of the same disc. The increased drag of a worn disc also tends to reduce the magnitude of the effect of air molecules. This is why a worn disc tends to fly slower (and a bit straighter) than a new version of the same disc; the increased surface drag reduces the overall dynamic fluid force.

Rough or textured surfaces tend to produce a greater turbulent flow and thus greater drag, but sometimes they actually decrease drag. This occurs when a layer of turbulent flow completely surrounds an object, and outside this turbulent flow a layer of directional, laminar flow forms. This is best seen in the flow created around the dimples of a golf ball.

Discs designed to throw and catch have a region of concentric, rough surface rings on the top sloping surface in an effort to reduce drag. As the air moves across the rings, flow transitions from laminar to turbulent flow. Drag is minimized because the airflow is connected to the surface as long as possible. Golf discs do not typically have dimples or concentric rings. Golf discs with dimpled or textured flight plates such as the Quest Defender, Gateway Diablo, and Latitude 64° Raketen attempt to take advantage of this airflow, although they have yet to be tested in a laboratory. Speed, as indicated by disc manufacturers, is a reflection of a disc's overall drag coefficient; the greater the speed rating, the less the drag.

The dynamic fluid force that acts perpendicular to the relative motion of a disc with respect to the air is known as lift force. For a disc to generate lift, pressures on the top of the disc must be lower than pressures on the underside of the disc. Lift force is caused by the lateral deflection of the air molecules as they pass over the flying disc. A disc exerts a force on the molecules that causes this lateral deflection, and according to Newton's third law of motion, the molecules exert an equal and opposite lateral force on the object. Lift force can be directed upward or downward and is most influenced by surface area and relative velocity of the disc.

The cambered shape of discs greatly increases their lift relative to a flat plate, and thus, even a disc thrown flat can develop appreciable lift. The flow of air over the top of a disc creates what is called a surface bubble on the leading edge of the disc, and this causes lift-producing suction; hence, even a disc thrown flat will tend to pitch up. The airflow under the trailing lip compensates for this pitching, which is why a disc seems as if it can fly forever before falling to the ground. Because golf discs have rim depth and camber (unlike a flat plate) and have a weighted circumference (most of the mass is located in the rim), pitching is significantly reduced during flight.

Although meaningful, a disc's lift-to-drag ratio can be misleading. For example, discs designed for putting tend to have low lift-to-drag ratios because of the significant amount of drag created by the rounded leading edge. Slight differences in rim depth, rim shape, or camber can have a significant effect on lift-to-drag ratio. A few millimeters difference in just one geometric component can have pronounced effects on flight characteristics.

Glide, as indicated by disc manufacturers, is a reflection of a disc's lift coefficient. Generally, the greater the glide rating, the greater the lift potential. Golf discs with deep rims and significant camber tend to have great lift potential. Golf discs of larger diameter (and thus with greater surface area) tend to have better glide potential than smaller discs. To meet the specifications approved by the PDGA, all golf discs must have a diameter between 21 and 30 centimeters. Throw-and-catch discs (such as the Discraft Ultra-Star) have much deeper rims than golf discs, and with a diameter of just more than 27 centimeters, they can exhibit excellent glide during flight.

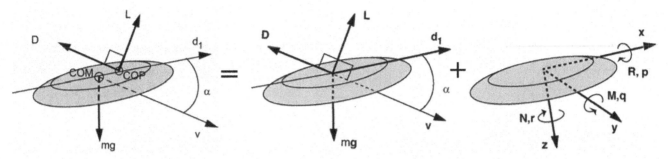

Forces and moments acting on a flying disc. The weight (mg) of the discs acts at the center of mass (COM) while the aerodynamic forces act at the center of pressure (COP). Drag (D) acts opposite to the velocity (v) as lift (L) acts perpendicular velocity (v). Roll (R), pitch (M), and spin (N) act at the x, y, and z axes respectively. *Figure by Sarah Johnson.*

Angles

Pitch angle (also called the **angle of attack**) is a disc's back-to-front tilt relative to its direction of flight. Pitch angle is an important variable because it is dictated by the thrower (initially) and because it significantly affects drag, lift, and other forces. The optimal pitch angle depends on the style of throw and type of disc, but nearly flat is a good reference point. A disc's side-to-side tilt immediately before release is called the throwing angle. As a disc flies, its side-to-side tilt can change significantly. The changes to both pitch angle and throwing angle during flight are what cause a flying disc's distinctive flight pattern. After all, golf balls do not fly in one direction and then another the way golf discs do.

Gravity, which is not dependent on pitch angle, throwing angle, or velocity, acts at a theoretical point on a flying disc called the **center of mass (COM)**. Because most discs have unvarying rim widths, the COM is located in the center of most discs. Some discs, like the Aerobie Epic, have an epicyclic rim and thus an off-center COM. Unlike most golf discs, the **gyroscopic stability** of the Epic depends on where the thrower grips the rim.

The flight dynamics of this type of disc have not been investigated.

Aerodynamic forces (drag and lift) act at a theoretical point called the **center of pressure (COP)**. Because the COP and COM are not in the same location, a moment is produced that causes a disc to spin (rotate) called pitch torque. The theoretical COP is not in the same location for every golf disc. Discs designed for shorter throws have a low rim-to–flight plate mass ratio. In other words, they have a weighted circumference, but the mass is fairly evenly distributed throughout the disc. These discs tend to have a COP close to the COM. Discs designed for longer throws have a higher rim-to–flight plate mass ratio. In other words, a greater proportion of their mass is located in the rim, and thus they have a COP farther from the COM.

Subtle variations in disc design, particularly the rim width and shape, can have pronounced effects on the distance between the COP and COM. It is important to note that COP is not a constant. As the pitch angle changes during flight, the COP moves accordingly. Basically, it is the forward and backward movement of the COP during flight that cause changes to the aerodynamic forces, which in turn impact a disc's dynamic flight characteristics. The image on page 93 illustrates the COM and COP of a disc in flight.

Gyroscopic Stability

Spin (also called rotation) has little influence on aerodynamics (drag and lift forces), but it does significantly impact a disc's flight characteristics. A disc thrown with little spin tends to wobble or flutter during flight, while a disc thrown with considerable spin will exhibit a more stable, predictable flight pattern. Imagine a spinning top. A gentle nudge will temporarily knock it off its spin axis, but it takes a much greater nudge to knock it over completely because spin adds gyroscopic stability. In much the same way, when a disc is spinning in the air, lift forces impact its pitch angle, but it will resist rolling (also called flipping). The gyroscopic stability that spin affords makes a flying disc amazingly resistant to angular motion, particular when it comes to rolling. The illustration on page 93 shows the roll axis (R) of a disc in flight.

One of the most intriguing facts about disc dynamics is that a flying disc will tend to maintain its spin rate even as it loses velocity. Spin rate relative to velocity is called the **advance ratio**. For example, a disc thrown right-handed using a backhand style of throw with appreciable spin and at a low pitch angle (nearly flat) tends to roll slightly, and thus its flight path will predictably turn to the right. As a disc loses velocity during flight, the subsequent increase in advance ratio significantly changes both its pitch angle and side-to-side tilt, and thus the impact of lift and drag forces. Toward the end of a disc's flight, its advance ratio will increase sharply as it loses loft and exhibits a right-to-left flight path (called **fade**). The degree to which a disc will turn and fade is largely dependent on its initial pitch angle, initial throwing angle, and the disc's design.

Choosing the Best Disc

The dynamics of a flying disc in flight are truly amazing. If you throw a disc at the optimal pitch and throwing angle, its flight pattern is inherently predictable; however, if you throw a disc just a few degrees off, the results can be embarrassing. Once you get accustomed to throwing a handful of discs, trying new ones is exciting, because subtle differences in disc design can produce significant differences in flight characteristics. Of course, understanding the basic dynamics of disc flight does not necessarily make you a better disc golfer, but it may help you in purchasing a new disc or choosong the right disc from your bag for a given throw.

Stability, as indicated by disc manufacturers, is a reflection of a disc's pitch moment and is rated on a continuum from overstable to understable. In theory, discs with a higher stability rating (at the overstable end of the continuum) have a greater potential to fly predictably during flight compared to discs with a lower stability rating (at the understable end of the continuum) because they are more resistant to rolling or flipping. However, when overstable discs lose velocity, their angle of attack changes rapidly, causing them to fade quickly. For a novice, overstable discs typically result in consistently poor (shorter) flight patterns because of this severe fade potential. Experienced players rely on the rolling resistance of overstable discs, and because they tend to throw with great initial velocity, their discs tend to fade much later in flight.

Stability is a tricky and ever-changing rating used by manufactures. Innova uses a two-variable stability rating (turn and fade potential) while Discraft uses a one-variable rating (essentially fade potential). We recommend Joe's Universal Flight Chart (gottagogottathrow.com) because it uses a more descriptive, two-variable rating. The variables are high-speed stability (HSS) and low-speed stability (LSS). HSS is the tendency of a disc to turn when it is flying fast early in flight, and LSS is the tendency of a disc to fade as it slows down later in flight. Also, Joe's Universal Flight Chart specifies a power rating for each disc. The power rating is the theoretical amount of force a player must generate to make each disc fly as it was intended. In general, we recommend beginners choose discs that are relatively low in both HSS and LSS. However, discs that are relatively high in both HSS and LSS can allow many novice players to take advantage of an *S*-curved flight pattern and the distance such a flight pattern affords. The ratings provided by both manufactures and universal flight chart designers are the results of their own field-testing and have not been independently scrutinized. Flight charts are very useful guides and nothing more.

Disc manufacturers are in the business of selling discs. They release new discs to keep the disc-buying public interested, and new drivers with greater speed ratings tend to sell well. However, speed does not indicate how far a disc will fly; rather, it is a reflection of how fast it can fly based on its profile drag. If you cannot generate significant force, then you are not likely to throw a disc with a slightly higher speed rating much farther than you would one with a lower speed

rating. Drivers can fly about 12 percent farther than midrange discs and about 21 percent farther than putt/approach discs, but drivers are highly sensitive to divergence from optimal release conditions. In essence, drivers can fly farther but are harder to throw accurately. Designing discs that can travel farther for people with limited power, skill, or experience may have as much to do with glide as speed.

If you are still working on the proper mechanics and you cannot generate a great amount of force, we recommend choosing a disc with excellent glide potential. In general, greater glide potential can lead to greater distance for the average player. Glide can be a tricky variable to determine, and some universal flight charts do not even report it. Manufactures are constantly trying to produce discs with better glide (while still maintaining stability) to appease both novices and professionals. Discs with higher speed ratings may sell well, but glide is the real magic of many discs. That said, we recommend carrying at least one disc for short throws with very poor glide potential so it can fly for a short distance and then fall to the ground, preferably in or near the target.

Types of Plastic

The type of plastic used in the manufacturing process can significantly impact the flight characteristics of a disc. Disc manufacturers use different polymers (essentially blends of plastics) during the manufacturing process, each with its own unique characteristics. Some blends even glow in the dark for evening play. Many manufactures have started using an **overmold** process that uses one type of blend for the rim (essentially for enhanced grip) and another for the flight plate (to improve durability). Expense can be a variable to consider, as the most expensive blends (or a combination of blends) cost roughly twice what the least expensive ones do. Greater cost typically equates to greater durability and, in some cases, greater stability during flight. The most basic blend (e.g., DX, Pro-D, or 300) is the least expensive and provides very good grip, but this blend tends to wear rather quickly. Because we want some of our midrange discs to wear a bit over time, and thus fly a bit straighter, we choose this blend for one of our "go-to" discs, and we always carry at least two: one slightly roughed up and one very roughed up from normal wear.

At the other end of the spectrum in terms of expense are blends that offer excellent durability (e.g., Champion, Elite-Z, or 400). These discs tend to retain their original flight characteristics better than any other blend. Because of this characteristic, we carry a few discs of this blend for use on holes where hitting a tree is likely. We would throw more of these types of discs, but we find them to be rather slippery when wet. There are, of course, blends that try to offer the best of both worlds in that they have very good durability and good grip (e.g., ESP, Star, or 400G). If you want your drivers to be durable (and thus fly consistently over time) and if you do not want to sacrifice too much grip, we recommend using this type of blend for drivers. Some manufacturers offer only one type of plastic in their drivers, and they all tend to feel and fly like this blend. Another type of blend offers excellent grip and a flexible, rubbery type of feel (e.g., R-Pro, Elite-X, or 300Rx). Because players want putters to have excellent grip and chain-grabbing flexibility, we recommend this blend of plastic for putters.

Some manufacturers offer only one or two types of plastic blends, and they all tend to feel and fly similarly.

A newer type of plastic blend incorporates tiny air bubbles into the plastic (e.g., Blizzard, Opto Air, or AIR). This blend is primarily used for drivers. The motive behind this new blend is relatively simple. Drivers are designed with wide rims and thus low profile drag. Wider-rimmed drivers tend to be heavy (150 to 175 grams) and thus require greater force to achieve maximum velocity. By infusing air bubbles into the plastic blend, wide-rimmed drivers can be made lighter (130 to 145 grams) and thus easier for beginners to throw with greater initial velocity. Some people contend that infused air allows for a greater rim-to–flight plate ratio. For more information about types of discs, please check out the manufacturers' information in appendix B.

Different Discs for Different Folks

If you are just beginning to play disc golf, we suggest you start by playing with a few discs. Consult the flight charts and ask knowledgeable folks at your local store or reputable online retailer for suggestions. Choose a putter, midrange, fairway driver, and driver, and stick with them until you learn how to throw them reasonably well. Finances aside, there is no reason to rush out and purchase 20 or more discs. Borrowing a friend's disc for a few throws is also a good way to test one out before purchasing. Some stores (like Disc Nation in Austin, Texas, and the Throw Shop in Ypsilanti, Michigan) will even let you demo discs before you purchase them.

More than choosing the best disc for the maximum distance, disc selection comes down to choosing the best disc for a given type of throw. As you hone your skills and learn different types of throws, you will undoubtedly start to carry more discs. The best disc for a **backhand throw** is not necessary the best disc for a forehand throw, and the best disc for an expert may not be the best choice for a beginner. While playing, disc selection ultimately comes down to where you want your disc to come to rest. In general, we recommend throwing an understable disc to a downhill target, because fade will be exaggerated, but some folks may deviate from that strategy. In addition, beginners may want to choose a more overstable disc in the wind to take advantage of fade potential. Principally, disc choice is dependent on several variables that we will discuss in upcoming chapters. Learning to throw different discs using a variety of throwing styles is a key part of learning to play the great game of disc golf.

Commonly Asked Questions

While advanced players might enjoy deep investigations into the dynamics of disc flight, most novice players simply want to know how to throw a disc straight and far. We will discuss throwing techniques in upcoming chapters, but as they relate to disc dynamics we will (at least partially) address a few of the most common questions beginners ask in this section.

"How do I throw a disc straight?" First, choose a disc rated by the manufacturer at the understable end of the continuum. We recommend choosing the slowest disc possible (as indicated by its speed rating) that is capable of reaching your intended target. If you have yet to acquire the skills needed to throw a driver with consistency, choose a disc designed for midrange throws or a putter. Next, try to throw the disc relatively flat and with considerable velocity and spin. If you throw it correctly, the disc will roll a bit early in flight, then fade slowly and finish fairly straight. This method will work when using either a backhand or forehand style. The idea is to choose a disc and throwing angle that does not penalize minor errors in throwing execution. Since angles will change during flight, you cannot expect every disc thrown perfectly flat will result in a straight flight. Overstable discs will fade, and understable discs will turn (at least slightly), even when thrown perfectly flat.

"How do I throw a disc far?" As mentioned previously, choosing a disc with a higher speed rating does not mean you can throw it farther than a disc with a lower speed rating. If you want to throw a disc far (for maximum distance or range), the most critical variables are throwing angle and initial velocity. As you grip a disc in your hand, it has a velocity of zero. The basic idea is to accelerate the disc though the throwing motion. Remember, acceleration is the rate of change in velocity. Creating a significant change in velocity requires a significant force to be applied over a distance. Distance in this case is the amount of limb displacement (or movement in space). For example, if you throw only using your wrist, you are able to exert a force on the disc using only a small amount of displacement. If you use your hips, shoulders, elbow, and wrist, the potential overall displacement is much greater. Using hip and shoulder rotation also increases the amount of musculature you use, and thus you can generate greater force. If you have long limbs (perhaps your friends refer to you as "lanky") then you have been blessed with some built-in displacement.

Optimizing force production results in the disc leaving your hand with maximum initial velocity. Accomplishing this feat is no easy task and is dependent on several variables that include individual variations in musculature and limb length. The timing of this kinematic (limb movements relative to each other) and **kinetic** (force production) **chain** of events is critical and takes a lot of practice. Immediately after a disc leaves your hand, gravity begins to pull the disc to the earth's surface, and the disc loses speed. After all, discs (unlike airplanes) do not have the means to gain velocity once they leave your hand. Any disc thrown with greater initial velocity is capable of flying farther, assuming drag, lift, and angle of attack are constants. If you have shorter limbs, then you have to make up for less potential displacement by timing the chain of events perfectly to maximize torque and ultimately velocity. In essence, timing is the most critical variable for most people and most throws.

"What about the weight of the disc?"
Remember, weight is a measure of the force of gravity acting on a disc. When manufactures talk about the weight of a disc, they really mean mass, and it is often measured in grams. Given that Newton's second law of motion is expressed as *force = mass x acceleration*, the sum of forces acting on a disc divided by its mass is equal to acceleration. Acceleration is inversely proportional to the mass. Thus, two of the same discs with differing weights will experience the same dynamic fluid forces, but the more massive one will experience less acceleration. In essence, using a lighter disc means you can use less force to achieve maximum instant velocity. Choosing the best weight ultimately comes down to personal preference. Because it takes less torque to throw a lighter disc than a heavier one, throwing two discs of varied weights the same way could, theoretically, change your release point. Future research might examine the effect of disc weight on release point and other variables in the **kinematic chain**.

Part III

The Skills of the Game

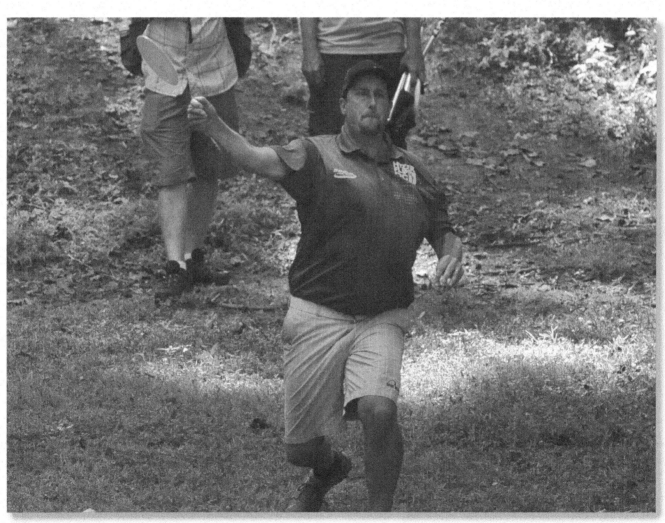

Brian Schweberger has one of the best thumbers on the professional tour. *Photo courtesy of PDGA Media*

Chapter 8

Backhand Throws

The majority of disc golfers, both amateur and professional, choose the backhand as their go-to throw. If you are a beginner, it is essential for you to learn how to throw an effective backhand if you aspire to play well. For many people, the backhand throw comes naturally. If you have tossed throw-and-catch types of discs at the beach or park, you have probably already self-selected a backhand throwing style.

Basic Grips

It is amazing how many different grips can be used to execute a backhand throw with accuracy and consistency. The key to determining which grip to use for a backhand (or any other type of throw) is to first accept that hands and fingers come in many shapes and sizes. The best grip largely depends on the length of your fingers, size of your palm, size of your thumb in proportion to your fingers, and length of your fingernails. Regardless of grip type, your goal should be to achieve stability and leverage. Your grip should feel stable, in that it is not likely to change during the throwing motion. More fingers on the rim of the disc may give you

a mechanical advantage when it comes to force production (more levers equals more leverage), as long as it is not at the expense of a clean and consistent release. Without a precise and consistent release, it is nearly impossible to consistently throw at the desired pitch and throwing angle.

The two most common grips used for backhand throws are the three-finger grip and the **power grip**. Either of these grips can allow you to achieve stability and leverage while throwing the disc. Make sure that your grip on the disc is firm but not tense. It is important that you do not try to grip the disc too firmly, because you will put tension on your hand, which may lead to the dreaded **grip lock**. This occurs when you grip the disc past the desired release point. In general, the firmer you hold on to the disc, the harder it is to let go. Some grips (particularly the power grip) lend themselves more to grip lock than others.

To execute the three-finger grip, put your fingers (minus the pinky finger) on the inside rim of the disc (see the photo on page 102). Notice how the fingertips are firmly placed on the inner rim of the disc. Players rest their fingertips in different ways on the inside disc rim, depending on the size,

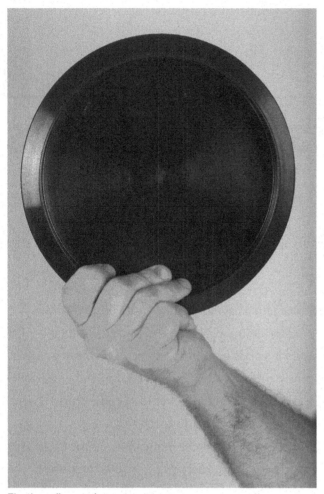

The three-finger grip. *Photo courtesy of Ryan Bumgarner*

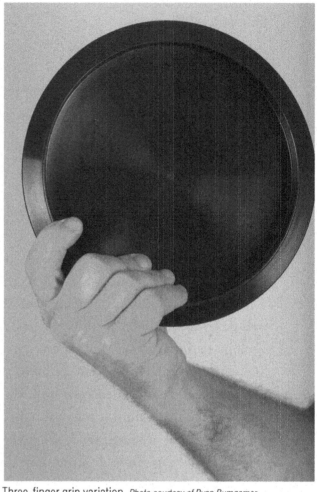

Three-finger grip variation. *Photo courtesy of Ryan Bumgarner*

width, and length of their fingers. Regardless of fingertip placement, the fingers are always curled underneath the rim. Your index finger should not be placed on the exterior portion of the disc rim.

If you want to achieve more stability, try placing your index finger away from the ring and middle fingers slightly. The index fingertip is still placed on the inside rim of the disc, but the edge of the disc lip will lie perfectly in the first crease line of the index finger (see photo above right). This slight variation in index finger placement may lead to more grip stability and throwing accuracy, although you will likely sacrifice distance. This grip is often

used for throwing throw-and-catch types of discs. Again, we suggest you avoid placing your index finger on the exterior of the rim.

To maximize potential throwing distance, most players choose to use a power grip. This grip is similar to the three-finger grip, but the pinky finger is also placed on the inside lip of the disc. Some players place their fingertips so they are touching the corner of the inside lip where the flight plate of the disc meets the rim (see opposite, left). Other players will place their fingertips on the inner edge of the rim, so the tips are not actually touching the inside corner or the flight plate of the disc. When

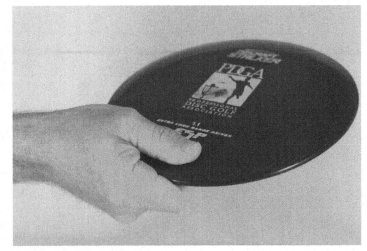

Flat thumb placement. *Photo courtesy of Ryan Bumgarner*

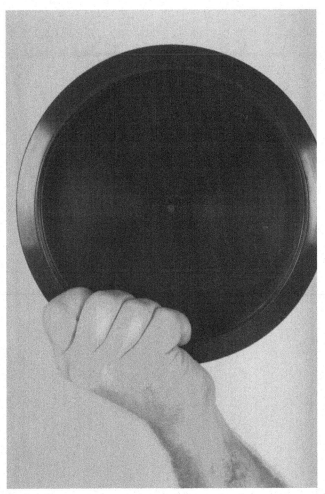

Power grip. *Photo courtesy of Ryan Bumgarner*

rock climbers are able to hold on with all four fingers, they call it a bomber grip because their hold on the rock feels bombproof. The power grip tends to have this feel—stable and powerful.

When executing either the three-finger or power grip, place your thumb on the top of the flight plate (see above right). Again depending on thumb size and comfort level, there are many different variations on how to use your thumb. Most players will lay their thumb completely flat, while others will flex their thumb so only the tip is touching the flight plate of the disc. Still others will lay the upper portion of their thumb on the disc and leave

the lower part of the thumb (near the knuckle) in the air. The differences are subtle but substantive. When throwing for maximum distance, we prefer to place the entire thumb with a portion of the palm on the top part of the disc. Regardless, the thumb's main purpose is to help stabilize the disc in your hand. Generally, you increase stability in the grip the farther you move your thumb toward the center, but you maximize distance by keeping the thumb near the outer portion of the rim.

The **fan grip** is very popular with players who have large hands and long fingers. We have seen this grip used mainly for approach shots, or by players who can throw extremely far. They often regulate their power by using a fan grip when inside 350 feet. The fan grip, or some variation of it, tends to be used a lot when putting. This grip is an easy one for beginners to learn because of the stability it provides.

Fan grips are achieved by fanning the fingers out on the underside of the flight plate of the disc (see image on the next page). Generally, the index finger stays on the rim so that the disc rests in the first crease line. Some players place the index fingertip

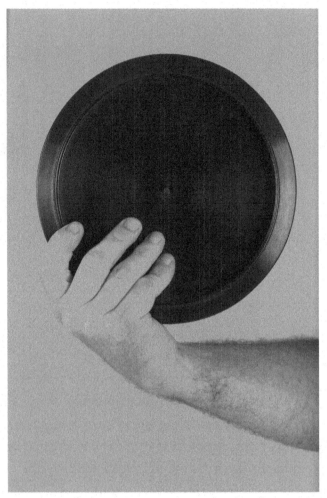

Fan grip. *Photo courtesy of Ryan Bumgarner*

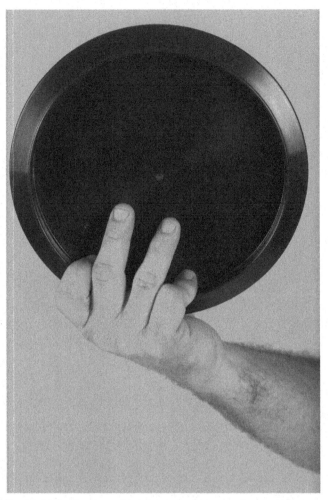

Double bird grip. *Photo courtesy of Ryan Bumgarner*

on the inside corner or underneath the disc where the flight plate meets the rim. The other fingertips rest underneath on the flat part of the disc (or fan out), which is why it is called the fan grip. We find we achieve the most accuracy and consistency when throwing approach shots or short drives if we tuck the index finger around the rim and then fan the middle finger and ring finger on the flat part of the disc. The pinky finger does not touch the disc at all. You will notice that the middle finger and ring finger are side by side, with a portion of the ring fingertip placed on the inner lip of the disc. Some

players prefer to rest the exterior portion of the rim on their pinky finger.

Other Grips

A variation of a fan grip is what we call the **double bird grip** (above right). The double bird grip is achieved by placing both the index and pinky fingertips on the inside of the disc rim. The middle finger and ring finger are then fanned out on the interior flight plate, pointing toward the center of the disc. In this grip, the index and pinky fingers serve as leverage and the middle and ring fingers provide stability. When executed properly, this grip creates remarkably strong leverage while maintaining stability.

Another backhand grip is called the knuckle lock, but it is more commonly known as the **Bonopane grip**. This grip is achieved by placing the rim of the disc in between your index and middle finger, so your index finger rests on the flight plate and your middle finger is tucked underneath the rim (see photo at right). The middle fingertip and the other two fingertips are placed on the inside corner of the rim, similar to the power grip. This is a difficult grip to master, and if you did not learn this grip as a beginner, we would not recommend switching to the Bonopane grip.

Throwing Angles

Remember, throwing angle is a disc's side-to-side tilt and is largely dependent on the alignment of your hands, arms, shoulders, and spine. A hyzer throwing angle is achieved when the outer rim of the disc (the one opposite your hand) is tilted downward. As you might expect, subtle variation (even a few degrees) can result in significant differences in a disc's flight characteristics. Backhand hyzers are generally easy for beginners to throw. Remember, nearly all thrown discs have a tendency to fade toward the end of flight, and a hyzer throwing angle will accentuate this fade. Discs at the overstable end of the continuum will fade significantly, while understable discs will fade much less. If you are just beginning to play disc golf, we recommend choosing understable discs to avoid all your throws "dive bombing" to the ground. The adjacent image illustrates a backhand hyzer throwing angle.

Technically, a hyzer is a throwing angle and not a type of throw; however, if you add a prefix or suffix, it becomes a type of throw. For example, a **hyzer flip** is achieved when you throw a disc at a hyzer angle and it flips (rolls or turns) significantly

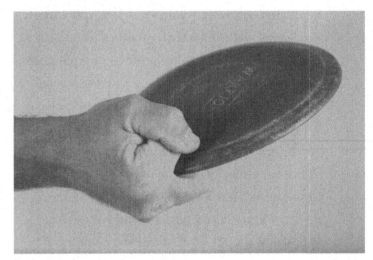

Bonopane grip. *Photo courtesy of Ryan Bumgarner*

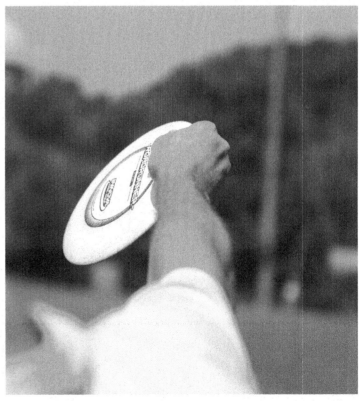

Backhand hyzer. *Photo courtesy of Cyndy Caravelis*

during flight and then finishes fairly straight. The amount of hyzer you need to put on a disc depends on the disc's stability. A hyzer flip is most often thrown using a very understable driver. If you throw a very understable disc with significant velocity, you will have to release it with a severe hyzer angle or it will roll too much. A **spike hyzer** is achieved when you throw an overstable disc at a severe hyzer angle high in the air in an attempt to make it fade quickly, thus the *spike* part. A spike hyzer that partially embeds in the ground upon landing is often called a **tombstone**. A Latitude 64° Scythe tends to work well for a spike hyzer, but the choice is ultimately up to you. With some practice, throwing backhand hyzers is fairly easy to learn.

An anhyzer (also called an annie) is the opposite of a hyzer. It is a throwing angle in which the outer rim of the disc is tilted upward. Again, subtle differences in throwing angle can result in significant differences in a disc's flight characteristics. An anhyzer throwing angle resists the natural spin of the disc and will often result in a disc that turns (rolls or flips) during flight. If you throw an overstable disc on an anhyzer angle, the result is a snake-like disc flight that initially turns, then fades (also called an **S-shot**). Understable discs thrown at a severe anhyzer tend to keep turning (or **flexing**, as it is often called) and will turn so much they hit the ground and become rollers. Anhyzers are fun for players of all abilities to throw because of the unique flight patterns that can result from trying different discs at various angles. The image below illustrates an anhyzer backhand throwing angle.

Biomechanics of the Backhand Throw

Proper throwing mechanics are critical to gain accuracy, consistency, and distance. As with any dynamic system, there are many components that must work together to achieve the desired result. The mechanics of the backhand throw include feet alignment, **reach-back**, **pull-through**, shoulder and back placement, release points, and the follow-through. We will first discuss how to throw from a standstill. We strongly recommend that you learn to execute a backhand throw from this fundamental position before you attempt to throw using a run-up (often used when driving from a tee pad).

Stance

Similar to a traditional golf stance, when you are lined up to throw, you should look straight down at your feet to get an idea of the flight line of the disc. In traditional golf, players will often place a club on the ground so the shaft is touching the endpoints

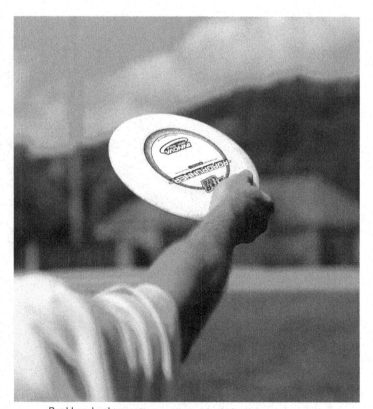

Backhand anhyzer. *Photo courtesy of Cyndy Caravelis*

of their toes. In this way, the club functions as an arrow pointing toward the intended target. When performing a backhand throw, this perpendicular stance alignment is similar to the basic stance used in traditional golf. Place your feet about shoulder width apart. Your toes should be pointing on a line roughly perpendicular to your intended target or flight line. Unlike throwing a baseball or softball, your front (lead) foot should be on the same side of your body as your throwing hand (technically called **ipsilateral** or **homolateral**). If you are right-handed, for example, your right foot should be your front foot.

Reach-Back

The next key phase is called the reach-back and is accomplished when you extend your throwing arm behind your body and away from the intended line of flight. Keep your shoulders about level, and reach the disc back to about shoulder height or slightly below. The more you reach back, the greater the potential initial velocity of the disc on release, and thus the greater the distance potential. The less you reach back, the less likely you are to miss your intended flight line. Ultimately, you have to weigh the advantages and disadvantages of greater arm extension. If you are attempting a

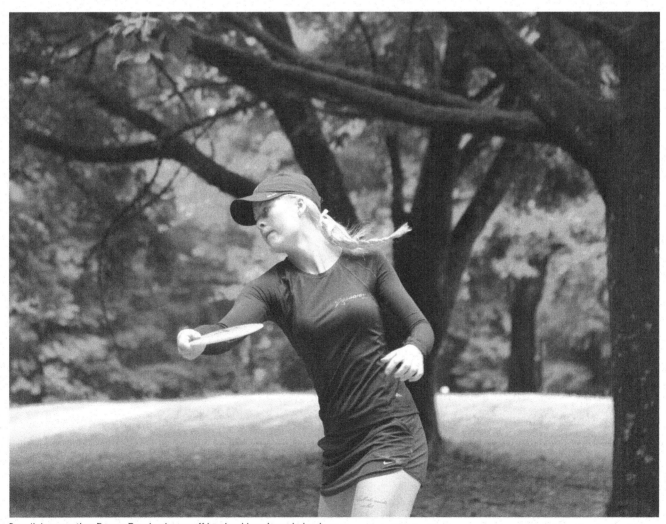

Swedish sensation Ragna Bygde shows off her backhand reach-back. *Photo courtesy of Prodigy Discs*

short-range throw, you do not have to reach full extension. Experienced players fully extend their throwing arm when they want to throw the disc as far as possible. Perfecting the reach-back takes a lot of practice and experience, but there are a couple common errors you should avoid.

Avoid grabbing the disc with your non-throwing hand while reaching back. Doing so will likely put your body in poor position. Lowering or "dipping" your non-throwing shoulder while reaching back will result in an upward throwing motion. Your disc will likely fly high up in the air (at a steep angle relative to the ground), and you will miss your intended line of flight. You will also likely release the disc on a hyzer throwing angle, whether you intend to or not. We call this very common throwing error the dreaded loop de loop. At the same time, dipping your throwing shoulder while you reach back may cause your throwing arm to be higher than your shoulders. The result is a disc released in a downward motion that can end up hitting the ground soon after release; hence this error is called a worm burner.

Front Foot Pivot

As you are performing the reach-back, you should execute a front foot pivot. The pivot of the front foot (on the ball of your foot) is an often overlooked but critical part of the backhand throw. When your front foot pivots away from your intended target, you are able to freely wind (rotate) your spine and load your hips. The rotation of your hips and spine is partially dependent on the amount you pivot your front foot. For a right-hander, the pivot foot is the right foot, and it rotates counterclockwise about 5° to 180°, depending on how far the righty is trying to throw.

Your toes will end up pointing away from your intended target. Your hips can then be sufficiently loaded and ready to provide the torque (rotary force) needed to propel the disc with substantial velocity. If you have played traditional golf, tennis, baseball, softball, or other sports, then you are likely familiar with the concept of loading your hips. Avoid lifting your front foot entirely off the ground. Instead, pivot on the ball of your foot at the base of your big toe. You will likely lose your sight line to the target (the major disadvantage of the backhand throw), but by loading your hips this way, you will be able to generate a great deal of torque.

Pull-Through

The pull-through phase is achieved by pulling the disc from the end of the reach-back to the release point. You should attempt to flex your throwing arm at the elbow joint and bring the disc close to your body during the pull-through. Allow your forehand to lag behind your upper arm. Your upper arm, forearm, wrist, and disc should form an *L* shape as you flex then extend your arm at the elbow joint. Keep the disc close to your body and maintain a stable wrist and forearm. Imagine pull-starting a lawn mower, chain saw, or small outboard motor, and you have the right idea. In essence, you should create a long lever arm during the reach-back phase, and then create a short level arm during the pull-through phase. Experienced players bring the disc close to their chest, particularly when driving.

Follow-Through

The follow-through is the final phase of the backhand throw. The momentum caused by the follow-through should naturally cause your entire

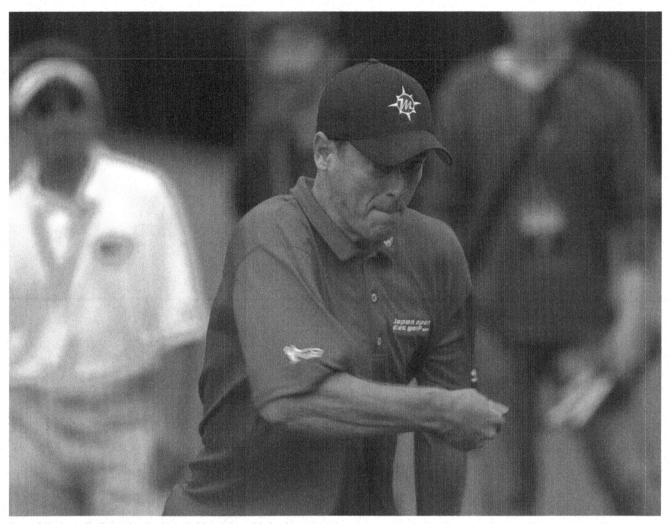

Barry Schultz pulls through a backhand drive tight to his body. *Photo courtesy of Innova Champion Discs*

body to spin a bit after you release the disc. Some folks contend that you can create more leverage at the release point if you lock your front foot in place as you are pulling through (much like keeping your front foot planted in the ground when playing traditional golf). We believe this strategy is potentially dangerous, as it can place stress on the knee joint. As such, we recommend that once you release the disc, you should allow your body to spin so that your left arm (for right-handers, and vice versa for lefties) comes all the way around, creating a 180° pivot.

As your throwing arm finishes toward your intended target, avoid focusing on significant wrist extension. This is a common misconception when executing a backhand throw. Snapping your wrist can put spin on the disc, but it will likely decrease the amount of velocity you can generate. Instead, you should feel the disc "pop" out of your fingers as if it had no choice but to release from your grip. Some people call this action tendon bounce. If you perform this technique properly, you may hear an audible snapping sound as the disc releases from your fingertips.

Executing a successful backhand throw takes a great deal of timing. In traditional golf, the saying is "Hips before wrist," and this concept is also true in disc golf. After the reach-back phase, begin your throwing motion by first rotating your hips, and let your shoulders and arm pull though the throwing motion. Imagine cracking a whip in the air or casting a fly-fishing line. As the whip or line moves through the air, the segments closest to the pole begin to move first toward the intended target. To get the disc to maximize acceleration through the throwing motion, you must start with your hips and allow your shoulders to rotate and arm to extend smoothly and quickly.

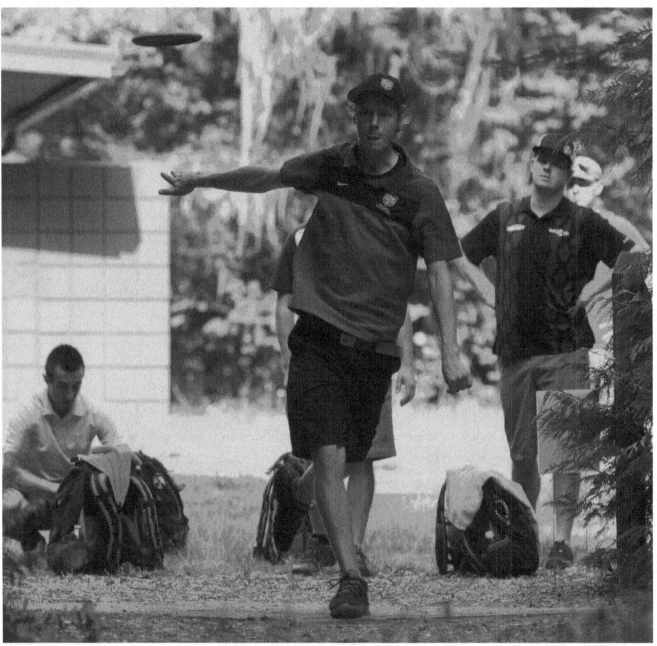

World distance record holder (863.5 feet) and trick shot phenom Simon Lizotte has a silky-smooth backhand follow-through. *Photo courtesy of PDGA Media*

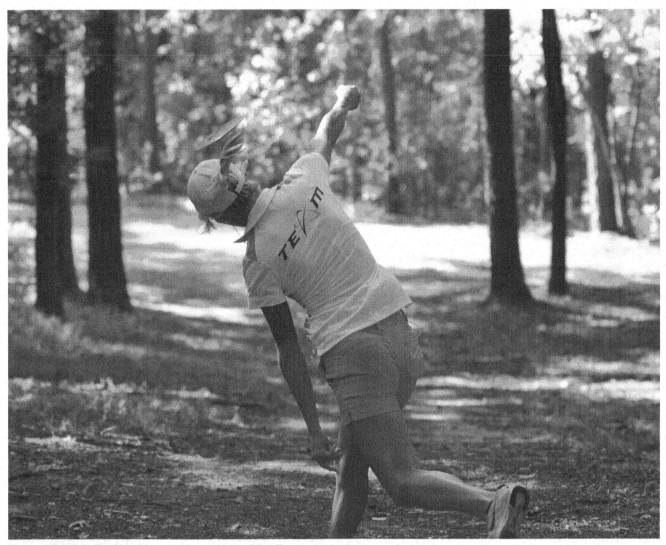

Catrina Allen rips a backhand hyzer with proper shoulder alignment. *Photo courtesy of PDGA Media*

Shoulder and Back Alignment

The alignment of your shoulders and back (and thus your center of mass) is critical to executing a backhand throw. Proper alignment of the back and the shoulders depends to a large degree on your intended throwing angle. A hyzer is easiest to execute when your shoulders are slightly in front of your waist and your center of mass is over your front foot. The more your center of mass is over your front foot, the greater the angle of your shoulders and upper body in relation to the torso and the hips. Beginners tend to find hyzer angles easiest to execute

because the body will naturally lean forward as a disc is thrown. To create less of a hyzer throwing angle, maintain your center of balance directly over your feet. Straight throws are achieved when your shoulders are level and your back is relatively straight. Your spine may be slightly flexed.

To release the disc at various hyzer or anhyzer throwing angles, you should tweak your stance a bit my moving your back foot to help align your back and shoulders. To help create a hyzer angle, place your back foot a few inches in front of your pivot foot (away from your body and in front of

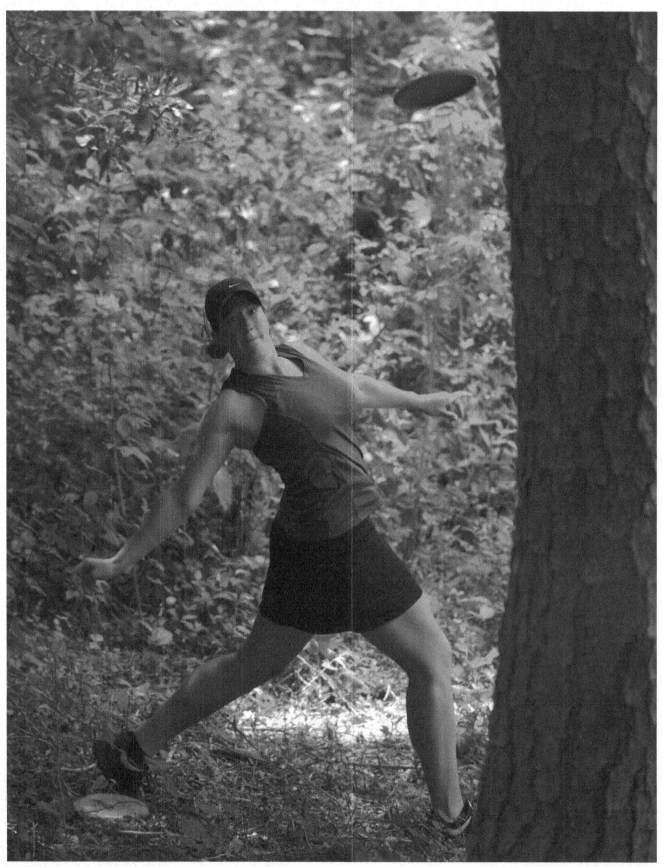

Val Jenkins opts for a backhand anhyzer. *Photo by Ryan Bumgarner*

your center of balance). This will allow for greater forward body lean without falling on your face. Your spine may be slightly flexed. For an anhyzer throwing angle, place your back foot behind your pivot foot (underneath your body, or behind your center of mass.) This will allow for greater backward body lean without falling on your butt. Your spine may be slightly extended.

An anhyzer throwing angle can be challenging for beginners to master. To release the disc at an anhyzer angle, your shoulders should be aligned slightly behind your torso and your center of balance should be more over your back foot. Your throwing hand will be a bit lower than your elbow and shoulder. The further your shoulders are behind your waist, the greater anhyzer angle you will be able to achieve.

The X-Step

If you have the space to make a run-up, you can throw a disc farther than from a standstill. Of course, executing any type of run-up takes more practice, and the timing of the throw becomes even more critical.

The **X-step** (and the **two-step approach**, which we will talk about later) requires coordination and timing. The goal is to get your body in the throwing position, as if you were throwing from a standstill, with some momentum toward the target. You could do a series of cartwheels if you wanted, but you have to end up in the basic standstill position if you want to throw accurately and consistently. In essence, you can accelerate the disc through the throwing motion better if you do not have to start from ground zero.

The X-step might seem complicated, but after some practice, we find that even beginners can execute it. The basic idea is the same for any sport skill that requires throwing with power (e.g., pitching a baseball). The key is loading your hips and allowing the implement (in this case, a disc) to accelerate through the throwing motion. After you try it a few times, it may help to say "left-right-left-right" to get the tempo correct.

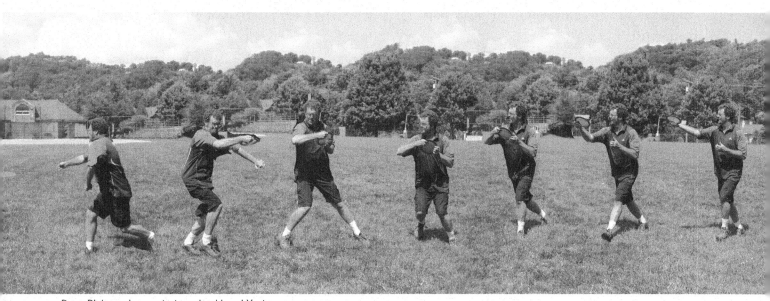

Ryan Pickens demonstrates a backhand X-step. *Photo by Cyndy Caravelis*

1. Start with your knees slightly flexed and your feet a little narrower than shoulder width apart.

2. Take a short setup step with your left foot (right for left-handers). Your upper body should remain fairly still.

3. Take a longer step with your right foot (left for left-handers) toward your intended target. Begin to reach up and back with your throwing arm.

4. Cross your left foot behind your right foot (the *X* part). This will allow you to rotate your spine as you load your hips, turning them away from the target.

5. Take a longer (plant) step with your right foot toward the target as you begin to transfer your weight forward. The placement of this step is critical.

6. Open your hips, followed by your shoulders. Pivot on the balls of your feet so your toes point away then move toward your intended target. Keep your throwing elbow bent so you create a short lever arm.

7. As your shoulders continue to unwind, keep your elbow tight to your body and allow your arm to extend toward the target. The disc should be ejected from your hand as you pop your wrist.

8. As you follow through, your shoulders should continue to rotate, as should your arm and hips, pivoting on your plant foot.

If you want to get even more power during the X-step, try the following:

1. Make sure your toes are pointing at least 180° away from the target as you load your hips. Practice pivoting your feet past the 180° mark, ensuring that you are maximizing spinal rotation.

2. Use a longer plant step toward the target. When timed correctly, this can increase the amount of forearm lag and thus increase the amount of torque you can generate.

3. As you follow through, make sure your body rotates (unwinds).

When to Execute a Backhand

Once you learn to execute the basics of throwing a backhand, success largely depends on choosing the right disc and throwing it at the optimal angle. Experienced players will choose a disc with the speed, glide, and stability characterizations needed to reach the target or intended landing area. Remember, both speed and glide will impact range (distance). Experienced players attempt to throw forcefully but smoothly rather than "back off the power" considerably. The backhand sets up well for several great types of throws that are fun to execute and thrilling to watch.

Generally, a backhand is great for a right-handed player to throw when the fairway bends from left to right (called a **dogleg** left in traditional golf on par-4 and par-5 holes), because a little hyzer and a little fade often results in a tidy left-to-right line of flight. For left-handers, the classic hyzer fade works equally well when a fairway bends from left to right (called a dogleg right in traditional golf on par-4 and par-5 holes). Anhyzer angles are a bit more difficult to throw, and because anhyzers tend to turn and glide, overthrowing the intended landing area is a fairly common mistake.

Backhand throws are best used when you face slight elevation changes and have lots of room for approach steps, unless you are using a standstill method. Because the backhand throw requires significant spinal rotation, it requires more movement of the body than other types of throws, especially when trying to achieve maximum distance. When you are using more of your body to execute a throw, there is more room for error, especially if the throwing surface creates a difference in height between your plant and rear foot. Subtle downhill throws also set up well for using a backhand.

If you are faced with a fairly level fairway that bends sharply from right to left (the opposite for southpaws) near the green or landing area (like an upside down J), then you might consider throwing a backhand spike hyzer. This throw is easy for beginners to learn because, as discussed earlier, hyzers are beginner-friendly, and most thrown discs tend to fade. Nearly every advanced player can throw a spike hyzer with success. When executing a spike hyzer, try using a three-finger grip or power grip.

To throw a spike hyzer, choose a disc at the overstable end of the continuum that will fade quickly and fall to earth on a steep hyzer angle. Release the disc on a steep hyzer angle and aim high. Your desired line of flight should be significantly elevated, anywhere from 50 to 150 feet depending on the open space available. If your throwing angle is steep, the disc might even tombstone by the target. Use caution when throwing to a green that slopes right to left or downhill. A spike hyzer that does not spike as much as you intended (and even some that do) can produce a disc that skips off the ground and away from the target (particularly on sloped greens). Spike hyzers are fun to throw because they are fairly easy to learn and a lot of discs seem to work well for them.

Another circumstance in which you should consider using a backhand is when you are trying to achieve the greatest amount of distance because of the torque the backhand technique affords. This can be accomplished through two types of throws, a hyzer flip and an S-shot. If you are a player who can generate at least a moderate amount of torque—or you are faced with a tightly wooded, straight fairway—consider giving the hyzer flip a try.

Disc selection is a key part of performing the hyzer flip throw correctly. Select a driver (or midrange disc with a high speed rating) that is very understable. Remember, seasoned and inexpensive plastics tend to be more understable. Set your feet to throw a big hyzer on release (about 40°), and try to throw it smoothly but with significant torque. Using a power grip seems to be most effective. The result should be a disc that quickly flips (rolls or turns), then flies relatively flat (or at a slight anhyzer angle) for a long portion of the flight. The disc should gain distance as it stabilizes and ultimately finish fairly straight or continue to turn slightly. If your hyzer angle is too great, the disc will not flip. Not enough hyzer, and the disc will flip too much and end up flying too far to the right (for right-handed players, and vice versa for lefties). Most professional players, with their massive torque and acceleration, do not use a hyzer flip and instead opt to throw a more stable midrange disc they can make fly straight. For the beginner or advanced player, hyzer flips are truly fun to throw and exciting to watch.

The other method we mentioned to achieve maximum distance, the S-shot, can be performed by players of all skill levels. Again, disc selection is important. Try using an overstable midrange disc

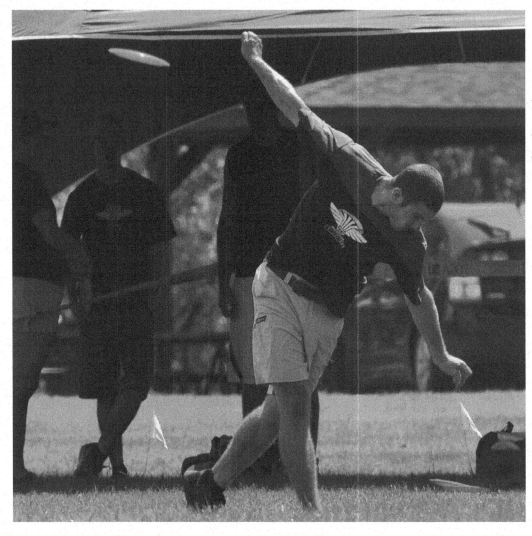

David Wiggins Jr., the former world distance record holder, dips his head to launch a backhand during a distance competition. *Photo courtesy of PDGA Media*

if you are a novice (remember, premium plastics tend to be more stable). This throw is executed by releasing an overstable disc at a steep anhyzer angle. The result is a disc that will first turn and then fade. The flight line will look like a swooping *S* in the sky. The significant time in the air spent turning, then fading, will often result in great distance. S-shots are best used when throwing on wide-open fairways, because they need a lot of room to work their magic. The S-shot is one of the throws that makes disc flight seem magical. After all, golf balls are not capable of flying one direction, then another during flight.

Right-handed players faced with a fairway that bends very tightly from left to right might consider using a backhand on an anhyzer throwing angle. The same is true for left-handers throwing right to left. In disc golf, very sharp doglegs are fairly common on wooded and partially wooded courses. The best disc to use for this throw, often called a turnover, is one stable enough to gently turn without rolling severely or fading at the end of flight. The keys to executing this throw are to keep your throwing shoulder above your non-throwing one, to get the anhyzer angle just right, and to make the disc work its magic. This throw takes a lot of practice to learn, but it is a venerable weapon in nearly every professional's arsenal.

Chapter 9

Forehand Throws

The forehand (also called a sidearm or flick) is an extremely valuable throw to learn. Although many right-handed players can make a backhand throw fly from left to right with success, it is just not the same as having an adept forehand in your arsenal. The forehand is executed by taking the disc with your throwing hand to the right side of your body (for right-handed players, and to the left for lefties) and then utilizing a flick of the wrist (technically called ulnar deviation) to throw the disc on the desired flight line. Imagine skipping a flat stone across a pond, and you have the general idea.

The forehand requires less overall body movement than the backhand, and thus the forehand throw has fewer potential error-causing variables. The other main advantage of throwing a forehand rather than a backhand is that you are able to keep your eyes on the intended target. Learning the basics of throwing an effective forehand will greatly increase versatility in your game and improve your chance for success on the course.

Basic Grips

Your forehand grip should feel firm but not tense. If you are squeezing the disc so hard that your hand hurts a little, you are gripping the disc too firmly. One of the most common grips for a forehand is what we call the **split finger grip**. When using this very stable grip, you may sacrifice some distance, but you should gain throwing accuracy. The split finger grip is executed by placing your index finger on the inner flight plate of the disc as it points toward the middle of the disc (see image on the following page). The middle finger is then split from the index finger, creating a *V* shape with the two fingers. One of the keys to a successful forehand grip is to make sure the fingertip of the middle finger is placed on the inside of the disc rim.

The other common grip is what we call the **unified finger grip** (also called a two-finger grip). This grip can help you create a bit more leverage than the split finger. Begin by placing your middle finger firmly on the inside rim and partially on the flight plate. Place your index finger closely beside your middle finger to create a

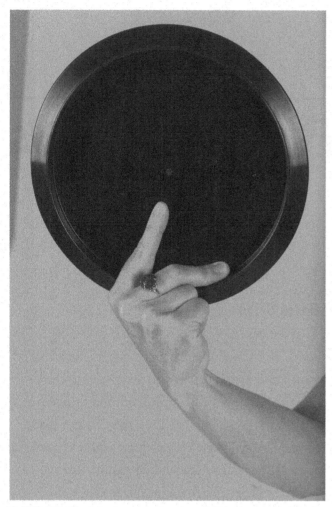

Split finger grip. *Photo by Ryan Bumgarner*

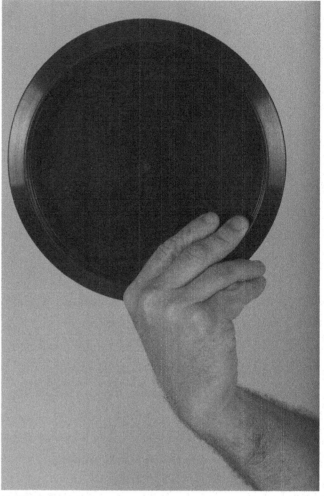

Unified finger grip. *Photo by Ryan Bumgarner*

unified feel. Place both fingers side by side on the inner rim of the disc so they are pointing in the same direction. For a variation that creates a little more leverage for some players, bend the middle finger inward at the first or second finger digit so there is more tension put on the rim of the disc. When you try using the split finger and unified finger grips, the following tips are important to keep in mind.

- The thumb is always placed on top of the disc, creating extra stability.
- The middle fingertip should straddle the interior disc rim and the inner flight plate.

- The ring and pinky fingers are used for support and stability.
- The exterior rim of the disc should be positioned in the corner of skin at the base of the index finger and thumb.

The first tip you should remember is that the thumb is going to rest on the top of the disc. It is important when you are throwing a forehand to push down on the disc with the tip of your thumb. This creates pressure between the thumb, the disc, and the two fingers on the inside, increasing stability and leverage. In actuality, the thumb is putting pressure on the top flight plate of the disc,

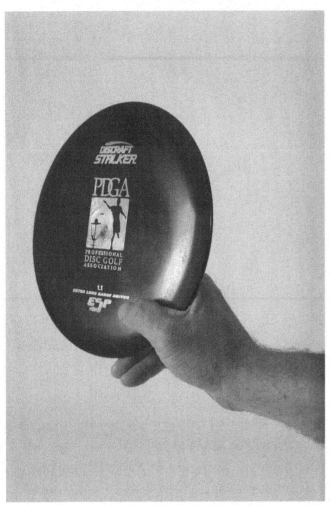

Thumb placement for forehand grips. *Photo by Ryan Bumgarner*

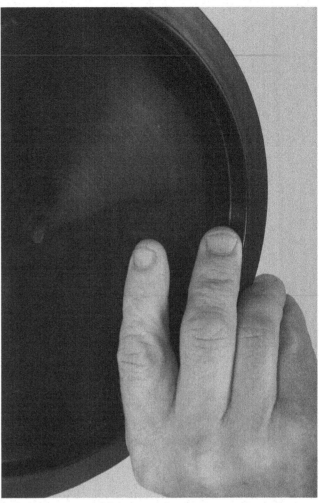

Middle finger placement for forehand grips. *Photo by Ryan Bumgarner*

while simultaneously your index and middle fingers are putting pressure on the inner flight plate of the disc. Ostensibly, you are holding the flat part of the disc between your two main fingers and your thumb. Some players will actually bend the last thumb knuckle so the fingertip of the thumb is pointed downward into the disc, creating even more pressure between the fingers and the thumb.

Another important tip for forehand grips is making sure the majority of the middle fingertip straddles the interior disc rim. Some players actually position the fingertip so it rests in the middle of the disc rim and the interior flight plate of the disc. Another way of thinking about this is the middle

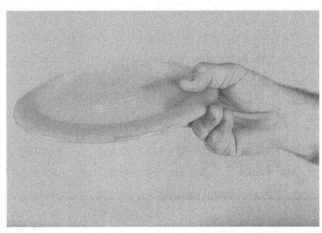

Ring and pinky finger placement for forehand grips. *Photo by Ryan Bumgarner*

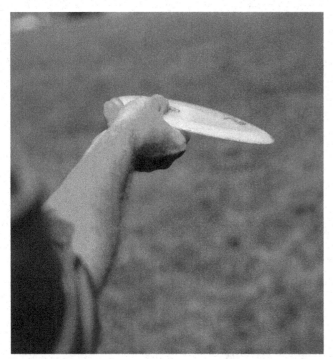

Forehand hyzer. *Photo by Cyndy Caravelis*

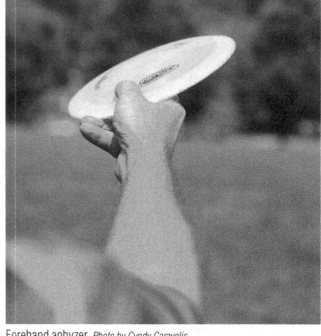

Forehand anhyzer. *Photo by Cyndy Caravelis*

fingertip straddles the inside corner that is created where the flight plate connects with the rim of the disc. This tip will lead to more accuracy while increasing leverage.

The third critical tip is to use the ring and pinky finger as extra support for the disc. It is extremely important that both these fingers are touching, adding necessary holding support for the disc. Basically, the bottom side of the disc rim will rest on these two fingers near the last section of your ring finger, depending on finger length. This will take extra pressure off your index and middle fingers while also providing more stability of the disc in your hand.

Finally, the fourth key tip is to utilize the corner of skin that is in between the index finger and the thumb as another resting place for the rim of the disc. If you were to place your right hand flat (palm side down) and put your thumb directly out from your hand, it would resemble a backward *L*. When gripping a forehand, the exterior rim of the disc is

going to be placed right in the corner of this *L* (the *L* shape will be lost once you have your fingertips and thumb tip in the proper place). It is important not to have any space between the exterior rim of the disc and the corner skin in between the base of the index finger and thumb. The more space you have, the less accurate and consistent you will be when throwing forehand.

Throwing Angles

Much like the backhand, a forehand hyzer is fairly easy to learn, and if you choose a disc at the overstable end of the continuum, it will fade much more than an understable disc. Both spike hyzers and hyzer flips can be achieved with a forehand throwing style. The image above left illustrates a forehand hyzer throwing angle.

Forehand anhyzers can be challenging to learn, but players with less power may find that they can maximize distance when executing this throw

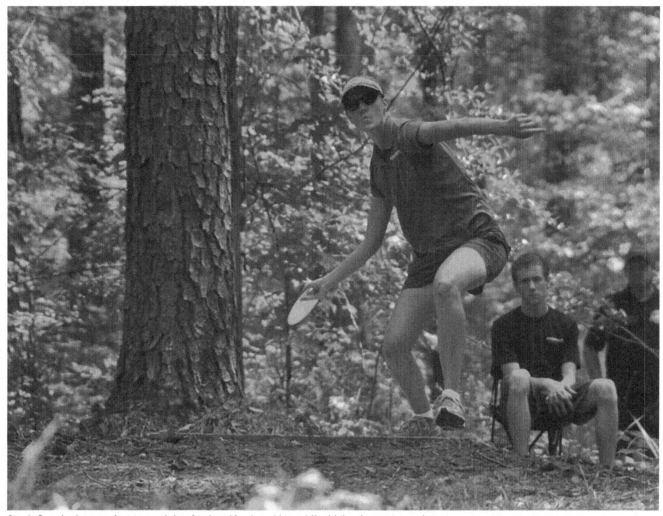

Sarah Cunningham prefers to reach her forehand back and low while driving from a tee pad. *Photo courtesy of Innova Champion Discs*

because of the *S*-shaped flight pattern created when using an overstable disc. The right-hand image on the opposite page illustrates an anhyzer forehand throwing angle.

Biomechanics of the Forehand Throw

As with all throws, mechanics are the key to gaining distance and accuracy. The basic idea is to accelerate the disc through the throwing motion. Acceleration is created with proper mechanics, and practicing the tips in this section will help you learn to throw 250- to 350-foot forehands pretty quickly. Once you understand how to throw with proper form, you will begin to throw with much less effort.

Stance

Much like the backhand, your feet should be about shoulder width apart (or a bit wider), and in line with your intended target. Your toes should be pointing on a line roughly perpendicular to your intended target or flight line. Unlike the backhand, your front (plant) foot should be the opposite of your throwing hand (called **contralateral**). If you

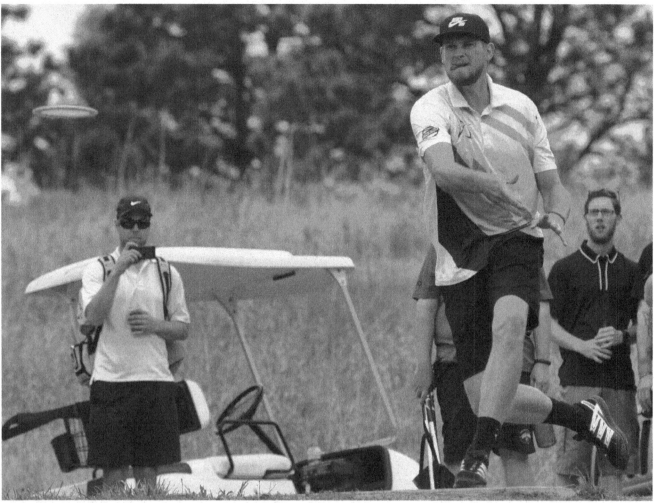

Spectators are treated to an impressive forehand follow-through from Jeremy "Big Jerm" Koling. *Photo courtesy of PDGA Media*

are right-handed, your left foot should be your plant foot. The heel of your plant foot may come off the ground a bit.

Reach-Back

Much like hitting a forehand in tennis, bringing the implement (a disc, in this case) back and to the ready position is critical. Start with the disc to the side of your body at about waist height. Rotate your spine and load your hips as you smoothly bring the disc back away from the direction of the target. Much like the backhand throw, the more you rotate your hips, spine, and shoulders, the more torque you can generate. The less you rotate, the

greater the control. The key is discovering the ideal amount of rotation for a given throw. Keep your center of balance over your base of support when performing the reach-back phase.

Keep the disc relatively flat as you bring it back and to the side of your body. Make sure your wrist remains stable, but it should cock backward (technically called radial deviation) like a springy hinge. This slight radial deviation keeps the disc stable in your hand and will add to the wrist pop before release.

Your shoulders should be fairly level, although your throwing shoulder may dip a little below your non-throwing shoulder. Keep your elbow joint below your wrist as you reach back. A common error occurs when the elbow moves away from the body during the reach-back phase. This can cause the disc to travel in an almost circular arc during the throwing motion. In tennis, a similar forehand motion is often called a *C* swing. We recommend a more compact, level reach-back, because the more error-causing variables you add to the mechanics of the forehand, the greater chance for errors in execution.

Front Foot Pivot

To ensure proper rotations, utilize a front foot pivot. Much like the backhand, your front foot should pivot clockwise. This aligns your body so your spine and hips can rotate freely. The more you pivot, the more you can rotate your spine and hips. Unlike the backhand throw, during the front foot pivot, you may not lose your line of sight on your intended target, unless you are using an X-step. This is one of the biggest advantages to the forehand throwing style.

Pull-Through

Like the backhand, the pull-through phase begins by rotating or "snapping" your hips to create torque. Allow your spine to rotate as your shoulders turn. As you pull your arm through toward your intended target, use your forearm as a leverage device. Keep your throwing arm elbow close to your torso so it acts like a large hinge. If your elbow is away from your body, disc acceleration may suffer. Allow your forehand to lag behind your upper arm. Imagine a bullwhip cracking in the air.

Follow-Through

Much like for the backhand, the follow-through is the final phase of the forehand throw. As you snap your hips, your arm should extend toward your intended target. The last part of this kinematic chain of events is unique to the forehand. Immediately before you release the disc, your wrist should flick forward (called ulnar deviation), which is why forehand throws are referred to as flicks. This subtle wrist motion is critical because it provides torque and allows the disc to spin freely. It may sound silly, but if you stand with your body completely still and only flick your wrist, the disc can fly 20 feet or more. As discussed, the position of your palm and wrist on release will partially dictate the throwing angle too. The momentum caused by the follow-through should cause your entire body to spin after you release the disc.

The key to learning forehand throwing angles is to focus on the rim of the disc. If the rim section opposite your palm is pointed upward (even slightly) on release, then the disc will begin its flight at a hyzer angle of attack. If the rim section opposite your palm is pointed downward, then the disc will begin its journey at an anhyzer angle of attack. If you want the disc to fly straight, you should release it fairly flat, which takes a lot of practice.

Shoulder and Back Alignment

For right-handers, if your right shoulder is lower than your left shoulder, you will have a greater possibility of creating a hyzer angle on the disc at the release point. And if your left shoulder is lower than your right shoulder, you will have a greater chance of achieving an anhyzer angle on the disc at the release point.

Keep your back relatively straight (spine neutral) and allow your shoulders to dictate the flight pattern. Engaging your core muscles (primarily the abdominals) will help keep your back straight.

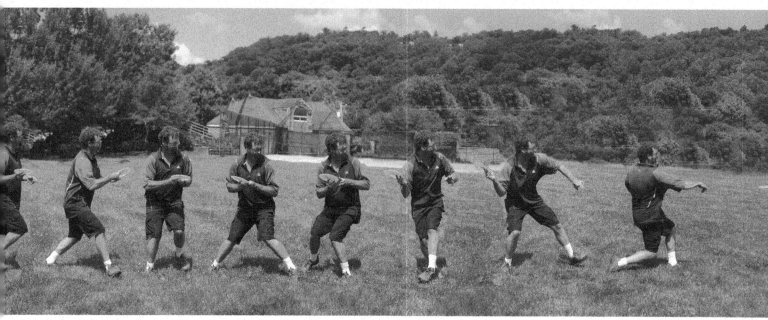

Ryan Pickens demonstrates a forehand X-step. *Photo by Cyndy Caravelis*

Make sure your shoulders mirror the angles present in the fairway. Whether you are throwing downhill, uphill, or traversing a diagonally angled fairway, you want to make sure your shoulders are parallel with the geometric line of the fairway. If you are throwing uphill, position your throwing shoulder slightly below your non-throwing shoulder in an attempt to mirror this line (remember: your non-throwing hand is in front for these types of throws). This tip will help you make sure your throw stays level with the ground.

Wrist and Palm Placement

To throw a forehand straight, keep your palm and wrist flat. Basically, your hand will be turned upside down with the disc resting flat on top of your palm upon release. To release the disc at a hyzer throwing angle, rotate your thumb down from this original flat-palm position, turning the hand slightly so your thumb is pointing more toward the ground. This slight movement of the thumb will help create the necessary disc angle upon release to achieve a hyzer angle of attack.

To release the disc at an anhyzer throwing angle, turn your thumb slightly upward from the original flat-palm position so your thumb is pointing more toward the sky. This causes the wrist and palm to rotate from the right to the left, creating an anhyzer release point. This slight movement of the thumb will help create the necessary disc angle upon release to achieve an anhyzer angle of attack.

It is easy to develop a bad habit of turning your wrist (technically called pronation) too far before release, turning the hand almost 180° from the flat-palm position so you no longer can see the palm of your hand. This exaggerated anhyzer release point will cause the disc to turn over (roll or flip) too quickly during flight. The key is to keep the palm of your hand visible while releasing the disc for the majority of forehand throws. Another way to think about aligning the release point up with the correct flight pattern for forehand throws is to think of your hand, thumb, and index finger as an imaginary gun. Ultimately, when you release the disc your index finger will be pointing in the direction the disc begins to fly.

The Forehand X-Step

Now that you know how to execute a forehand throw from a standstill position, we will discuss the most common method to use when driving a disc from a tee pad. One advantage of using a forehand throw is that you can create a lot of leverage with very little arm movement and body rotation. However, if you have the space for a run-up approach, you can throw a disc farther than you can from a simple standstill. Again, executing any type of run-up takes more practice, and the timing of the throw becomes even more critical. When driving from a tee pad, most players tend to use the unified finger grip. Some players will incorporate a little X-step or a large X-step to help their lower body get in proper placement. If you watch slow-motion video of the best professional players, you may notice many of them exceeding 270° of rotation when utilizing the X-step. For right-handers the forehand X-step unfolds as follows:

1. Take a short step with your right foot (left if you are a lefty) so your toe ends up pointing diagonally toward 1:30 (the target is at 12:00). This small step sets up the initial spinal rotation.
2. Take a step toward the target with your left foot as you reach the disc back.
3. Pivot your right foot so it is pointing away from the target as you rotate your spine. Your back should be turned slightly away, and your eyes may remain on the target.
4. Open your hips, followed by the shoulders. Pivot on the balls of your feet so your toes are pointing away from your intended target. Keep

your throwing elbow bent so you create a short lever arm.

5. As your shoulders continue to unwind, keep your elbow in fairly tight to your body and allow your arm to extend toward the target. The disc should be ejected from your hand as you pop your wrist.
6. As you follow through, your shoulders should continue to rotate, along with your hips, pivoting on your plant foot.

When to Execute a Forehand

Similar to the backhand, once you learn the fundamentals, learning to execute successful forehands largely depends on selecting the right disc for the job and throwing it at the optimal angle of attack. Experienced players tend to choose a disc with the speed and glide characteristics needed to reach their intended target, and they try to throw forcefully but smoothly rather than backing off the power substantially. The forehand sets up well for several throws that are cool to execute and inspiring to watch.

Typically, a forehand is a great throw for a right-handed player to use when the fairway bends from left to right, because a slight hyzer angle of release combined with fade during flight can result in a useful right-to-left line of flight. For left-handers, the classic hyzer fade works equally well when a fairway bends from right to left. Much like throwing a backhand, anhyzer angles are more difficult to throw, and because anhyzers tend to turn and glide, overthrowing the intended landing area is a pretty common mistake.

All the throws illustrated in the backhand chapter (spike hyzer, hyzer flip, S-shot, and turnover) can be performed using a forehand throwing style. In general, choose a disc that is more overstable than you would use for the same type of throw when using a backhand throwing style. In addition to keeping a line of sight to the intended target, using a forehand has other advantages (as well as a few disadvantages) over using a backhand technique.

In general, the forehand requires less overall body movement than the backhand, which tends to result in less overall torque. All the world distance records have been accomplished by people using a backhand style, and it is unlikely we will ever see a distance record set using a forehand. The vast majority of experienced players will use a forehand for distances ranging from 250 to 400 feet. A few professional players use the forehand style as their go-to drive and can throw a forehand more than 450 feet.

So even though forehands are not typically used for long-distance throws, there are some other opportune times to utilize them. The best situations in which to consider using a forehand style include:

- Little room for a run-up
- Unstable ground below your feet
- Throwing uphill or downhill
- Very tight bends in the fairway
- Narrow fairways
- S-shots

A forehand is excellent to use when you are faced with an unstable throwing area and a standstill throw is your best option. In these situations, when you do not have a lot of room for a run-up or when there are roots, rocks, or other obstacles interfering with your foot placement, try using a forehand. For many players, from absolute beginners to touring professionals, the forehand is simply easier to throw from a standstill than a backhand.

The forehand can also be an excellent way to generate power when standing on an incline. Using a backhand style on an incline often requires you to come across your body with your throwing arm, which often creates uneven body alignment on release. When throwing uphill or downhill from a tough stance, it is difficult to keep your shoulders parallel to the ground angle. When you choose to use a forehand style, you do not have to cross your body with your throwing arm. This helps ensure your shoulders and body are aligned properly with the angle of the hill. In particular, when throwing up a steep incline with no run-up, we encourage you to try using a forehand. Beginners are often amazed at the positive results.

The forehand drive is often a good choice for very tightly bending fairways when the intended flight line is similar to an upside down *L*. In these situations, you want the disc to fly relatively straight for about 100 to 250 feet then fade fairly quickly. A backhand anhyzer is more difficult to execute in this case, especially if the fairway does not have a lot of open space. The forehand is also a wise choice for narrow fairways. When using a forehand throwing style, very little body movement is needed to generate torque, and thus there are fewer potential error-causing variables.

Finally, using the forehand style is an excellent way to execute an S-shot that flies in the opposite direction of a backhanded *S* throw. In this context, we recommend choosing an overstable driver or fast midrange disc. The result is a disc that begins at an anhyzer angle of attack, then initially turns (or rolls), then fades later in flight.

Chapter 10

Overhand Throws

Overhand throws like the thumber and tomahawk are essential to have in your disc golf bag of tricks. Some players have a philosophical issue with these throws because the disc does not fly "as it was intended." Indeed, these throws will result in a disc that will often tumble (also called corkscrew) in the air rather than gracefully gliding. Performing the tomahawk and thumber is similar to throwing a baseball or softball, or serving a tennis ball. As such, former baseball, softball, and tennis players seem to take to using overhand throws with relative ease. Ultimate players call the tomahawk a hammer. Regardless of your background, learning to execute one or both of these types of overhead throws is well worth the effort.

Basic Thumber Grips

There are three basic ways to grip a thumber, all of which are illustrated in the images that accompany this section. One way to grip a thumber is to put your thumb on the inside rim of the disc with the outside rim resting on the very first crease of your index finger. Utilizing this crease will help secure the disc in your hand, which may lead to greater consistency and accuracy. For an alternative grip, place your index finger on the exterior of the disc flight plate, allowing the rim of the disc to rest in the first crease of your middle finger. This grip allows for a little bit more stability, especially if you have small hands or short fingers. Either way, the thumb should be placed on the inside rim of the disc.

Players who have large hands with long fingers often use the third-most-common grip for the thumber. For this grip, the thumb is still placed on the inside rim of the disc, but the creases of the index and middle finders are not used at all. Instead the fingers are curled into the palm of the hand (similar to making a fist) and the rim of the disc rests in the skin between the index finger and the thumb, similar to the forehand grip. If you have large hands and fingers, then the disc will rest securely between the thumb and the curled-up fingers. However, you will find that if you have small hands or short fingers, the disc does not have a lot of support when utilizing this thumber grip, and you likely will be better off trying one of the first two grips.

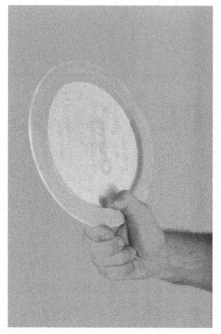
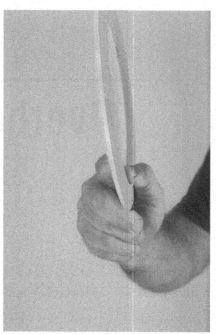
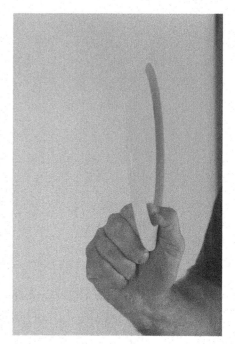

Thumber grips. *Photos by Ryan Bumgarner*

Basic Tomahawk Grips

The tomahawk grip (see photo, opposite) is much different from the thumber. It is very similar to the unified finger grip used to throw a forehand in that you place your index and middle fingers underneath the disc. The ring finger and the pinky finger also serve as support. A portion of the rim of the disc actually rests on your ring finger. Your thumb is also placed on the exterior flight plate of the disc. Similar to the forehand grip, this allows another part of the rim of the disc to rest perfectly in the skin between the thumb and the index finger (adding more support). Some players like to place their index and middle fingers on the bottom of the disc, while others put them on the inside rim. Either way, as with the forehand grip, both fingers should be placed side by side with no separation, or "unified" as we like to say.

Biomechanics of the Overhand Throw

When possible, your front foot (also called the lead foot) should be on the opposite side of your body as your throwing hand (called contralateral) and about shoulder width apart. If you are left-handed, your right foot will be your lead foot.

Stance

First, align your front leg with the target. Your front foot should be placed at an angle so the toes are not pointed directly toward the target. Next, find your center of balance and get in a stable, athletic stance.

Reach-Back and Front Foot Pivot

Once your body is set and your front leg is in line with the target, lower the disc down toward your waist, then smoothly reach your arm back behind your body. The farther you reach back, the greater the displacement and the greater the potential torque you can generate. As you reach back, rotate your spine and hips. Your shoulders should turn about 90°. Much like throwing backhands and forehands, pivoting your front foot will make loading your hips much easier.

Begin the throwing motion by "snapping" your hips. Raise the disc above your throwing shoulder (almost directly over your head) by smoothly flexing and extending your arm. Your legs should flex then extend as you throw. Generate some thrust with your non-throwing arm by bringing your non-throwing elbow toward the target and downward, just like throwing a baseball or softball. Utilizing your non-throwing arm in this way helps ensure that you will execute a proper follow-through. If done correctly, your center of balance should shift to your front leg and your back foot should rise off the ground. Avoid too much wrist flexion and extension. Instead, accelerate the disc through the throwing motion and let it "pop" out of your grip.

Shoulder and Back Alignment

When executing overhand throws, it is very important that your shoulders stay centered over the top of your body throughout the throwing motion. You will find it helpful to lower your throwing shoulder slightly as your body is turning away from the target and the disc is dropping below your waist. As you bring your throwing arm forward, you should then lower your non-throwing shoulder slightly. Your back should remain relatively straight while throwing overhands, and it is wise to engage the bottom half of your core by tightening your abdominal muscles as you are beginning the throwing motion. This will help ensure that your

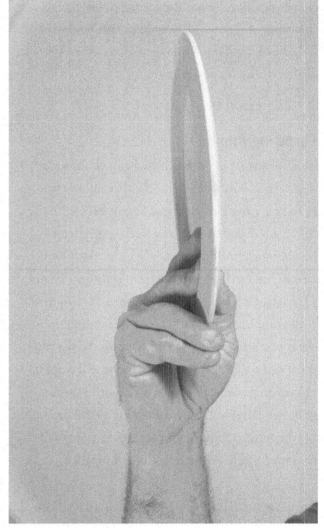

Tomahawk grip. *Photo by Ryan Bumgarner*

back stays fairly straight during the throw and will add stability to the kinematic chain.

The biomechanics of the tomahawk and thumber are very similar, but there are some important differences. The main difference (other than the grip) is the bend and curvature of the spine. To execute a tomahawk you should extend your spine a bit, which will naturally cause some body lean. Make sure your shoulders are behind your buttocks as you begin the throwing motion. This extension helps get your throwing hand in proper position before the release point. Of all the types of throws illustrated in this book, the tomahawk tends to feel the most awkward because of this throwing position.

Throwing Angles

Most of the time, when throwing a thumber or tomahawk, you will release the disc above your head at an angle of attack of about 40° to 60°. The result is a disc that flies at a steep angle before tumbling (or rolling repeatedly). For right-handers, a thumber tends to tumble from right to left and a tomahawk tends to tumble from left to right. This tumbling can vary greatly depending on the disc stability and throwing angle. Generally, the more stable the disc, the more it will tumble. However, some understable discs with excellent glide potential will only roll about 45° before flying nearly perfectly upside down. Determining which throwing angle to use takes lots of practice.

Driving from a Tee Pad

You can create a little momentum and thus increase your throwing distance by incorporating what is also known in baseball and softball as the **crow hop**. This can be executed on a tee pad or any relatively level lie if you have ample room to move. The crow hop is a type of X-step with a culminating leap, and it can actually help with timing the throw. To execute the crow hop, you should have at least five feet of space for a run-up. Like the forehand throw, overhand throws require a contralateral arm-leg action.

Begin with your left leg pointing in the direction of your target (at 12:00), with your toes pointed at 1:30. Then pick up your back (right) foot first and quickly bring it in front of your front foot. As soon as your back foot has begun to move forward, lift your front foot. It is important to note that both feet are in the air at the same time, which is why it is called a crow hop. The back foot turns sideways as it is in the air and lands facing 3:00. Your front

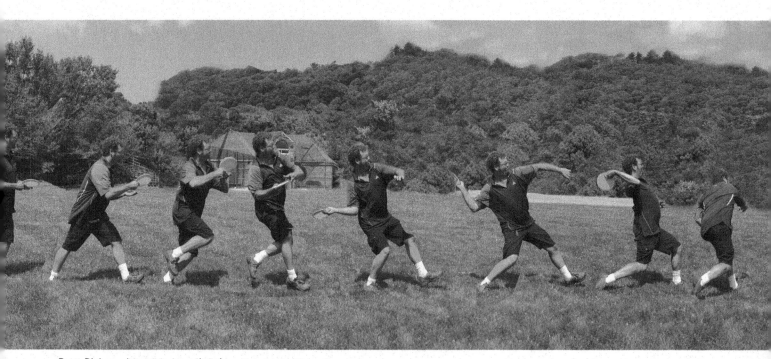

Ryan Pickens demonstrates a thumber. *Photo by Cyndy Caravelis*

foot rotates away from the target while in the air. Your toes should land at 4:30. At this point, your entire body will be turned away from the target and your throwing arm will have rotated about 210° away from the target, ready to uncoil toward the intended target. It sounds complicated, but with just a little practice, the crow hop is fairly easy to learn. The throwing sequence is illustrated on the opposite page.

When to Execute an Overhand

Some players think overhand throws are ugly to watch. We think they can be as exciting to watch as they are to throw. Some experienced players use an overhand as their go-to throw, while others simply use them as valuable short-range utility throws. They can be easy to learn and throw, but you should be extremely careful when throwing thumbers and tomahawks. When executing either of these throws, particularly when you are fatigued, it may be easy to injure your rotator cuff (a group of tendons and muscles in the shoulder connecting the humerus to the scapula). Thus, using correct technique and properly warming up for overhand throws is imperative.

Whether you decide to utilize overhand throws as your go-to throw or as a utility throw, they can be excellent choices to use in these situations:

- Island greens or greens with sharp drop-offs
- Uphill throws
- Heavily wooded fairways that bend in two directions
- When the greatest percentage of open space is over or through foliage

Because of the tumbling flight pattern often created with overhands, one of the best times to use a tomahawk or thumber is when you are faced with a green or landing area surrounded by out-of-bounds (such as island greens), or that has extremely steep slopes. Overhand throws tend to bounce more than skip when they hit the ground, and may give you a better chance of having a makeable putt. Unlike balls, discs do not bounce well. Bouncing overhand throws tend to be unpredictable, but they do not tend to bounce very far.

When faced with a steep uphill throw, try using a thumber or tomahawk. Although forehands tend to work well for uphill throws, they require your shoulder height to be close to parallel with the angled slope of the fairway. This can be hard to visualize and even tougher to execute. However, overhand throws do not require you to change your shoulder placement as much, and you can focus all your attention on the proper release. In addition to the easier body position, the flight pattern of the overhand is consistently more accurate when faced with steep uphill slopes. Overhands tend to gain altitude quickly in flight and then lose it quickly, looking as if they drop out of the sky. If the situation calls for it, try utilizing this unique flight pattern to your advantage.

Both tomahawks and thumbers work really well on zigzagging fairways that bend left to right to left or right to left to right. Densely wooded courses tend to have fairways with these multiple bends. These holes often set up best for an overhand throw because of the vertical flight pattern. Instead of throwing a traditional *S* pattern, you may be able to "cut the corners" by utilizing a relatively straight flight pattern that stays vertical. In essence, overhand throws tend to fly "straightish."

As discussed earlier, the throwing angle will vary significantly depending on the intended flight path and stability of the disc used. If your lie is surrounded by trees and you must navigate a very narrow and low gap, then you may want to release the disc at a very low throwing angle (about 15°). If you are trying to throw over a grove of trees that stand about 80 feet tall, you should release the disc at a steep throwing angle (about 75° to 80°). An overhand throw thrown at a 0° angle of attack (flat) can result in a disc that flies upside down before eventually tumbling (if at all).

If you are off the fairway and surrounded by trees, an overhand can definitely create more realistic alternatives to get back on track. When you are faced with a lie surrounded by trees (often called being in **jail**), the greatest percentage of open space may be above the trees or foliage. In this context, throwing a backhand or forehand may not be feasible. Plus, it is likely that the throwing motion for the backhand or forehand is obstructed due to low-lying limbs or bushes. The overhand throwing motion may allow you to get above these obstacles while throwing the disc back to the fairway. Sometimes your only option is to crash through dense foliage. Of course, this should be your last option, and it may require a unique type of thumber.

If you throw a thumber by lowering your throwing arm so that it comes down to the side of the body, you might be amazed at the results. The best way to visualize this motion is to picture a baseball player pitching a sidearm off the mound. The majority of baseball pitchers throw the ball by bringing their arm over the top of their body, as you would when executing a traditional thumber. There were some pitchers (such as the legendary Gene Garber from the Pittsburgh Pirates) who threw amazingly well with a sidearm motion. Sidearm pitchers drop their arm so it is nearly horizontal or lower as they reach back. They are still twisting their body in the same way, but instead of their arm coming over the top, it is lowered to the side of the waist, creating a different trajectory and spin on the ball. Well, the same is true in disc golf. If you lower your arm while throwing a thumber, you will find the disc flies low and with a tight, corkscrew-like pattern.

Many disc golf holes are designed with obstacles players must avoid, typically requiring flight lines that go to the left or right. The beauty of overhand throws is that you have the option to fly your disc over the top of these obstacles. You might be amazed at how well thumbers and tomahawks will make it over (and through) some pretty challenging obstacles. By not having to throw around obstacles, the unique flight pattern of overhand throws effectively shortens the distance to the target. Once you are comfortable throwing overhands, you can get in the habit of thinking about whether it is better to approach the target by going around obstacles or straight at the target by flying the disc high in the air and over obstacles.

Chapter 11

Rollers

A backhand or forehand throw designed to fly for a short distance and then land on the ground and roll like a wheel is aptly called a roller. Rather than flying in the air, rollers remain on the ground for the majority of the distance traveled. Generally the disc will hit the ground after about 70 feet or less. Rollers are most often thrown using a backhand style and, as you might expect, backhanded rollers will curve one direction and forehand rollers the other, depending on their handedness. Overhand throws can also be used to create rollers.

Basic Roller Grips

Fortunately, you do not have to learn a new grip to throw a roller. The grips used for rollers are generally executed exactly the same as you would any backhand or forehand throw. However, there is one type of power grip typically used for a backhand roller that tends to work quite well, especially if you have smaller hands (see the photo on page 134). Basically, when you place your four fingers underneath the rim of the disc, instead of touching the disc flight plate with the tips of your fingers, move them so they rest on the edge of the disc rim and are barely inside the disc rim.

Biomechanics of the Roller

The biomechanics of the roller are very similar to throwing a backhand or forehand on a steep anhyzer angle. The stance is the same, and the kinematic chain of events should begin at your hips. To throw a roller, you should drive your elbow toward the ground to get the angle right and pop your wrist to initiate spin. Your wrist should be completely open when releasing the disc (see the photo sequence on page 135). As we stated previously, discs "like to spin." Well, discs rolling on the ground have to spin, and greater spin usually equates to greater distance. Remember, drag, lift, and stability cannot be considered conventionally when a disc is rolling on the ground.

Throwing and Landing Angles

When throwing rollers, both the throwing angle and landing angle (the angle of the disc when it hits the ground) are critical. The optimal throwing

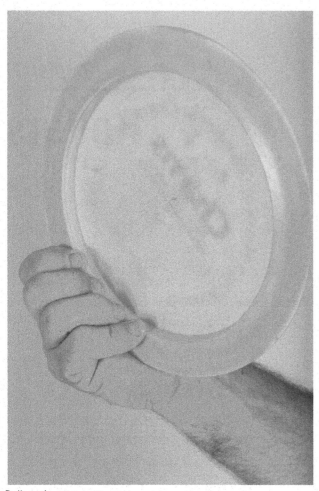

Roller grip. *Photo by Ryan Bumgarner*

of the disc. If the landing angle is 90° (called dead vertical), it will likely roll quickly to the right (when throwing a right-handed backhand). If you are throwing a forehand roller and land the disc dead vertical, it will very likely roll to the left (opposite of the backhand) because the disc is spinning counterclockwise rather than clockwise. Remember, if the disc lands dead vertical, it will likely curve and roll out quicker. A roll-out is when a rolled disc loses velocity and slowly comes to a stop. If the disc lands on a 45° to 60° angle, the disc may continue to roll on that line farther down the fairway until it flips to a vertical position and then slowly rolls to the right or left. It may sound complicated, but it just takes some practice to see which angle is most effective.

When to Execute a Roller

Disc selection is critical to throwing an effective roller. Many experienced players will use a very seasoned, "flippy" disc and release it on a hyzer angle. The result is a disc that quickly flips to an anhyzer angle of attack before it hits the ground. However, some players will use more stable discs because, when thrown properly and with significant velocity, they tend to roll straighter and farther. For example, when throwing right-handed, a backhand roller with an understable disc will tend to roll to the right. The same throw with an overstable disc will tend to roll to the left.

Whether you decide to utilize rollers whenever possible or as an "only when necessary" utility throw, they are an excellent choice to use in the following situations:

- Gaining extra distance
- Diagonal hillsides

angle for a successful roller depends on your goal—maximum distance or scrambling out of a tough situation. Also, the best throwing angle has a lot to do with the disc you have chosen to throw and the direction of the wind. Generally, you want the disc to land on a 45° to 60° angle when it hits the ground. If the disc on the ground were represented on a clock, it would be pointing to between 10:30 and 11:00 for thrown backhands and between 1:30 and 2:00 for forehands, assuming you are right-handed.

It is important to understand that landing angle will greatly influence the rolling direction

- Tight alley shots
- Low ceilings
- Corkscrew fairways

When driving from a tee pad, rollers are best used on long, flat fairways where the target exceeds the maximum throwing distance you can reach in the air. It is very important to scan the fairway and make sure it is free of fallen trees, roots, tall grass, and small swales. Any of these obstacles, even though they may seem minor, can greatly influence the roll, even when the fairway seems flat. Rollers that travel in the wrong direction can be disastrous. We have often seen older players use rollers when driving for maximum distance. We think of rollers as a very "cognitive" throw, in that getting the throwing angle, landing angle, and disc selection right is collectively more important than throwing with the velocity of a professional player.

Fairways that feature dramatic angles can be excellent places to use roller drives. If you are faced with a fairway that has a diagonal angle and you have to traverse a hillside, a roller could be the best way to get to the target. These fairways have diagonal angles, with the target on the right. This is a perfect place to throw a right-handed backhand roller (if you are right-handed) because, if thrown correctly, it will turn over and curve right up the hill. You are also more likely to keep your disc in bounds.

Both backhand and forehand rollers can be excellent to use in scramble situations when you need to get out of an extremely tight alley in the middle of the trees. If you do not have any open space above you, look along the ground to see if there is a landing area where the disc could begin to roll out of the woods and back in the fairway. Many times you will find a narrow **route** out of jail. Of course if you find yourself in trees, it is unlikely you will have a lot of throwing room, so generally you will be executing a forehand or overhand roller upshot.

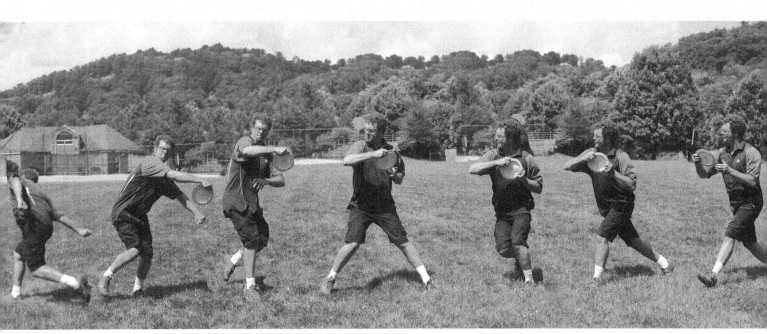

Ryan Pickens demonstrates a roller. *Photo by Cyndy Caravelis*

Forehand rollers are a lot easier to execute standing still with very little room. Backhand rollers require a lot more mechanical movement of the arm when throwing, while the forehand roller can be executed with just a flick of the wrist and can still have a range of approximately 100 feet when thrown properly. The roller can also be a perfect choice in other unique situations when the target is surrounded by trees that are extremely hard to get around and there is no way over the top—a classic example of a low-ceiling green. Instead of trying to go through the tiny gaps or up and over the trees, a roller can allow the disc to go under the foliage.

Two other roller variations are called the **sky roller** and the **cut roller**. The sky roller is best defined as a throw that flies in the air about 180 to 250 feet before it turns over, hits the ground on a vertical angle, and begins to roll. It is executed by throwing a long anhyzer drive or using an extremely understable disc that, when thrown on a hyzer, flips over into an anhyzer. Experienced players who can execute sky rollers are capable of getting the disc to travel more than 500 feet. However, to throw a sky roller you must have a lot of open space. As you might expect, perfecting the sky roller takes a lot of practice.

The cut roller is executed by releasing the disc at an anhyzer angle. When thrown properly, it will roll in an upside down *U*-shaped pattern and are perfect for a corkscrew fairway. When faced with a challenging fairway, you can throw a cut roller on an anhyzer angle so that when the disc hits the ground, it rolls on that same anhyzer line. Of course, this can be very difficult to execute and takes a lot of practice to perfect. The forehand cut roller is thrown in a similar way except you are throwing it on the other side of the body and getting it to cut and roll to the right in an upside down *U* pattern.

In addition to the shape of the fairway, the factors you should take into account before choosing to throw a roller are the strength of the wind and the type and condition of the grass. If there are huge wind currents coming across the fairway, a rolling disc is going to go drastically off course, more so than if you threw it in the air. Rollers have the best results on non-windy to slightly windy days. Tailwinds and headwinds do not have much effect on a disc once it is rolling, but they will affect a disc while it is flying in the air. Tailwinds make turning a disc over into an exaggerated anhyzer much harder. On the other hand, headwinds will turn a disc over even quicker than normal.

The length, type, and dampness of the grass must also be taken into account. A lot of times you will be in a situation where there are some beautiful fairways for rollers and the grass does not seem that long, but in fact it is three to four inches in length. Of course, this will decrease the velocity of the disc as it rolls, which will decrease the distance traveled. If the grass is very damp, the disc will also roll much slower. If faced with any of these variables on the fairway, it may be wiser to choose an air flight pattern rather than attempting a roller.

Some players love to throw rollers, and others never attempt them. Rollers are definitely a situational throw that must be practiced to be perfected. Because drag, glide, and speed cannot be considered conventionally, even impeccably thrown rollers can hit an ill-fated weed or root and wind up rolling in the wrong direction.

In addition to some open-field practice, we recommend trying rollers when playing casual rounds with friends. Sometimes, when faced with the greatest adversity (such as a lie surrounded by thick foliage), throwing a cut roller from one knee is your only chance to advance the disc. In situations such as this one, having the ability to throw a roller can save your round from the brink of disaster. Some experienced, older players enjoy the challenge of taking what the land gives you and getting maximum distance for getting it right.

Chapter 12

Putting

As the old saying in traditional golf goes, "You drive for show and putt for dough." This is also true in disc golf. After all, a 450-foot drive and a 20-foot putt are both counted as a single throw on the scorecard. Even more so, missing short-range putts can be extremely frustrating and can trigger a negative attitude on the course. This is especially true when you outdrive your competitors on a given hole but end up scoring worse because you missed an easy putt. Understanding the keys to successful putting and spending a lot of time practicing will shave strokes off your score and help keep your mental game in a state of flow. Putting skills can be improved late in life, and as discussed in chapter 1, it is easy and inexpensive to set up a disc golf putting green in your backyard or local practice area.

When it comes to putting, your primary objective should be to develop a consistent style and routine that minimizes error-producing variables. Tweaking your go-to putting style and trying different styles in different situations is part of the learning process. Practicing different styles will ultimately help improve your go-to style and help create versatility in your game. As discussed

throughout this chapter, regardless of which style you choose, you should always remember the four fundamentals of good putting: balance, aim, weight transfer, and follow-through. There are three types of putting stances (in-line, straddle, and staggered) and five basic putting styles (spin, pitch, loft, turbo, and flick). Each of the five putting styles can be executed from the three types of stances, although some styles seem to work best with certain stances. Some players use a comnination of styles (e.g., a "spush"—a combination of a spin and push putt).

Stances

When using an in-line putting stance, your rear foot is placed directly in line with both your lead foot (your right foot if you are right-handed and your left if you are a lefty) and the target. Your feet should be about shoulder width apart or a bit wider. Some players prefer to position their lead foot so their toes are pointing at the target, whereas others will point their tocs at about a 45° angle. Either way, the toes of your rear foot should point toward the target. Some players prefer to face their throwing shoulder to the target, while others

139

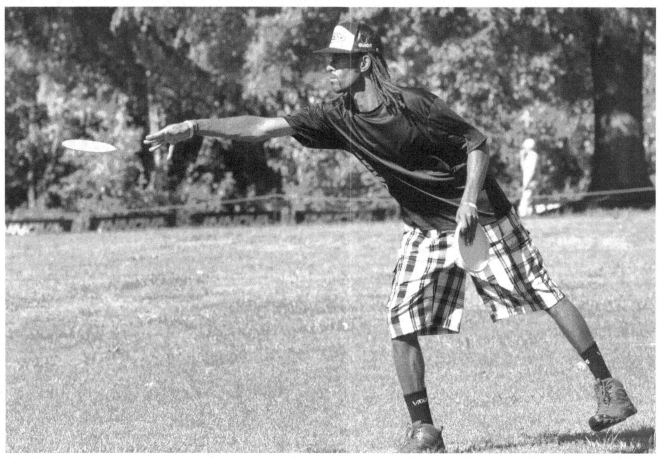

Philo Brathwaite's classic in-line putting stance. *Photo courtesy of PDGA Media*

choose to square their shoulders to the target. As you transfer your weight from your center mass to your lead foot, your rear foot will often come off the ground.

Even if you prefer to use an in-line stance, practicing a straddle stance is a good idea, because it allows you to step around trees or other obstacles. When executing a straddle stance, your shoulders should be square to the target and your feet should be placed on a parallel line (rather than in line) with the target. Excellent straddle putters often demonstrate a good bit of dynamic knee flexion and extension and tend to keep their back straight. When straddle putting, the disc is brought down to or below the knees to create the momentum needed

to propel the disc into the air. Oftentimes, if faced with a long putt, straddle putters will lower the disc almost all the way down to the ground. Many players prefer to use a modified straddle stance (one foot slightly in front of the other) called a staggered putting stance.

Spin Putt

By definition, a **spin putt** is a putting style that propels the disc on a relatively straight line with very little variation in loft. A spin putt is released from the hand with a good bit of velocity and tends to have a lot of spin, hence the name. Spin putts can be released on a flat hyzer or anhyzer throwing angle.

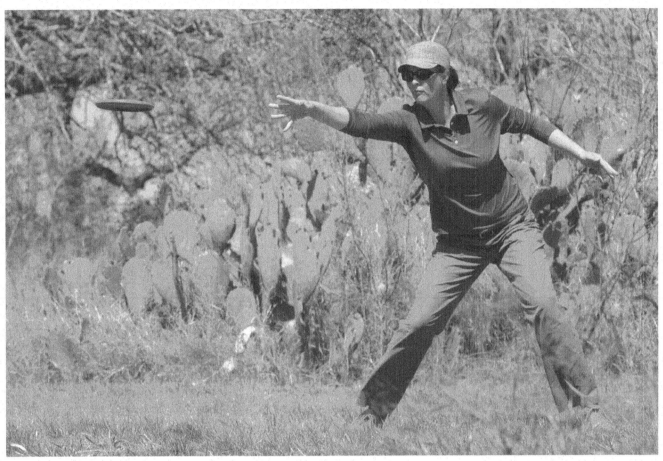

Des Reading's balanced staggered putting stance. *Photo courtesy of PDGA Media*

Different variations for the spin putt grip are illustrated in the photos on page 142. All four fingers should be tucked underneath the disc, utilizing the first crease on your index finger as a contact point for the bottom rim. Aligning the disc rim with this crease may increase stability of the disc in the hand and accuracy at the release point. The index finger should be tucked under the rim. The thumb should rest on the top surface of the disc for support, although it is rare that you will see players exert much pressure on their thumb while putting. Some players slightly fan their fingers versus keeping them all firmly on the inside rim.

To execute a spin putt, bring the disc back to your body on a relatively straight line by flexing your arm at the elbow. Your knees should be flexed. When pulling the disc back toward your midsection, your wrist should flex a bit. Your forearm should remain steady and firm as your wrist flexes. Extend your knees quickly but smoothly. When you release the disc, your arm and wrist should extend toward the target and produce significant spin on the disc. This wrist pop will create spin on the disc, which will tend to keep it on a straight line during flight. After all, flying discs are most stable and predictable when spinning. The most common mistake beginners make is aiming too low to avoid a long comeback putt. If you find you are missing low often, aim for the top of the target.

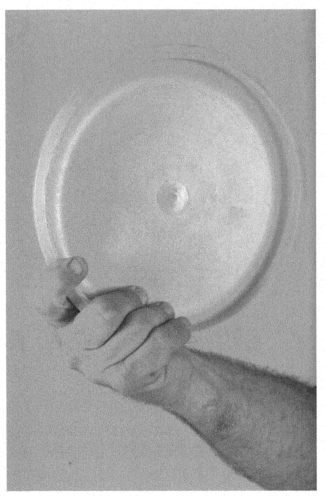 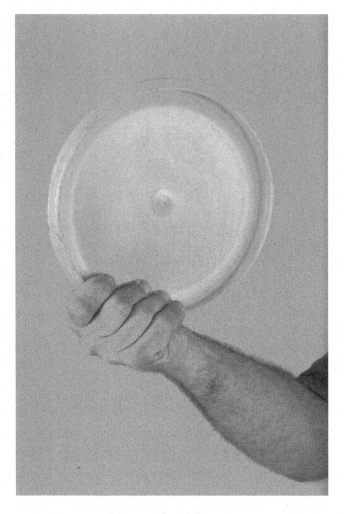

Spin putt grips. *Photos by Ryan Bumgarner*

Pitch Putt

Executing a pitch putt requires a significant amount of low to high arm motion (called shoulder abduction). Players that prefer to use a straddle stance will often begin the putting action by bringing the disc very low, nearly all the way to the ground. When using an in-line stance, most players prefer to start the putting action by bringing the disc to about waist level. Because of the low to high arm action, pitch putts tend to fly on a higher trajectory than spin putts, much like a pitch shot in traditional golf.

To grip the disc for a pitch putt, your index finger may be placed on the rim of the disc. Many players will fan out their fingers underneath the disc instead of having them tucked in tight on the rim of the disc. There are some players who prefer to keep their fingers on the inside rim while pitch putting. Because most players will use a fan grip, one tip that will ensure the disc flies on a moderately high trajectory is to focus on flexing your middle and ring fingers as you release the disc. As you release the disc, flex both fingers slightly to get a little extra push underneath the disc while it

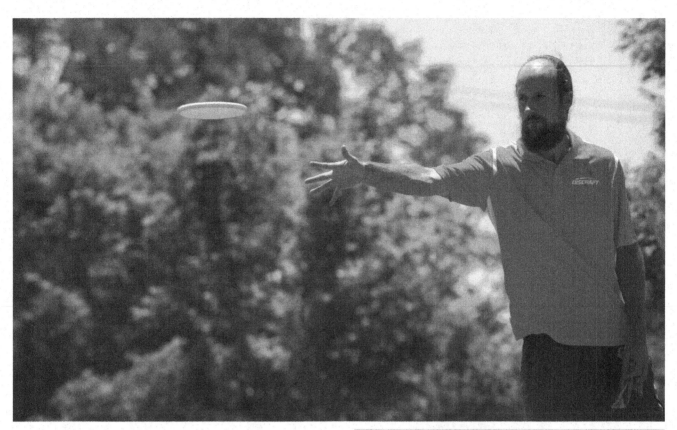

Michael Johansen uses an upright spin putting form. *Photo by Ryan Bumgarner*

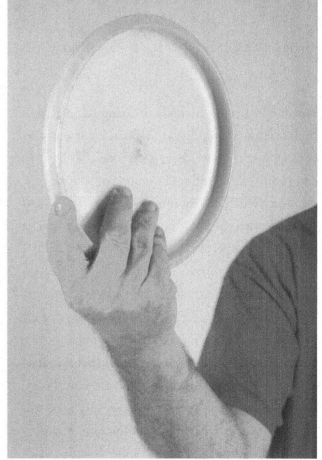

is leaving your hand. This may help you release the disc flat.

Pitch putts are most often released on a roughly flat throwing angle and are pitched up some. Pitch putting typically requires less wrist action and more leg action than spin putting. Rather than popping the disc from your hand, pitch putts require a more subtle—but still smooth—release. Avoid throwing the disc like you would if you were playing catch. When pitch putting from an in-line stance, push off the ground quickly but smoothly by extending your rear leg. From a straddle or staggered stance, extend both legs until you come up on your toes. When executing a pitch putt, it is best to aim a bit higher than you would for a spin putt, because the disc will lose loft during flight. The most common

Pitch putt grip. *Photo by Ryan Bumgarner*

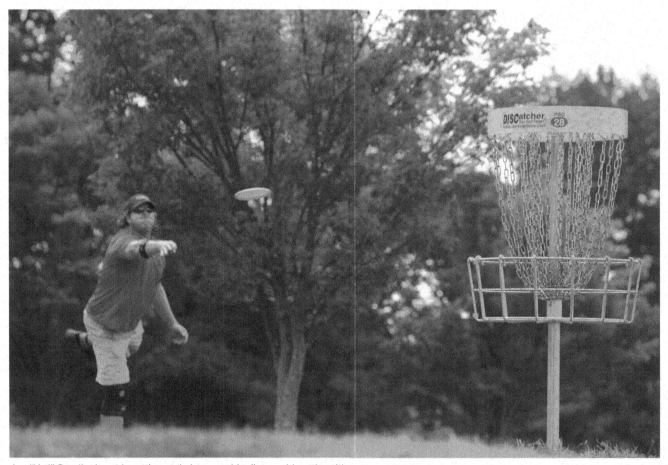

Jay "Yeti" Reading's push putting style has won him five world putting titles. *Photo by Ryan Bumgarner*

mistake beginners make is releasing the disc too high and on a steep hyzer angle in an attempt to compensate for a weak leg extension. Pitch putting can produce a significant amount of spin on the disc, which is why some players refer to it as "spitch" putting. Most professional players prefer to use some type of pitch putting technique.

Players large in stature may opt for more of a **push putt** because moving their center of mass a few inches can create a significant amount of force. Push putting is executed similarly to pitch putting, although the putting action dictates that the disc starts around waist height and not close to the ground. Most push putters produce very little spin on the disc. Rather than arm abduction, it is elbow extension that gives impetus to the disc. Because

flying discs are most stable when spinning, there are very few push putting purists.

Loft Putt

A **loft putt** (also called an **elevator putt**) can be executed with or without a great deal of spin. A loft putt is the rough equivalent to a lob shot in traditional golf. Rather than flying on a moderately high trajectory like a push putt, a loft putt flies on a sharply upward trajectory toward the target, then it loses loft rapidly as the disc drops in or near the target. If you have ever played a game of horseshoes, you have the general idea. Most players prefer to use a push-putting grip, or a subtle variation, when loft putting.

To execute a loft putt, align your legs and shoulders the same way you would when either spin or push putting. Next, while flexing your knees, lower the disc to about knee level while keeping your throwing arm relatively straight. Bring the disc to the release point by forcefully extending your legs while using an upward arm/shoulder motion (called shoulder abduction) to propel the disc upward.

Turbo Putt

Turbo putts tend to be more of a situational putt. It is very rare that you will see a player who consistently uses the turbo putt as his go-to putt. Turbo putters do have the distinct advantage of not having to practice either spin or pitch putts. By definition, a turbo putt is one that is released at or above your shoulders using your wrist and forearm to spin the disc.

There are two different types of grips that are commonly used for the turbo putt: the **longhorn grip** and the **four-finger grip**. The longhorn grip will be easy to master if you are a University of Texas fan; the grip resembles the hand symbol that UT fans use to show support for the team while saying "Hook 'em Horns." While using the longhorn grip, you want to place your pinky finger and your index finger on the rim of the disc while resting your middle finger and ring finger underneath the disc for stability. You should have two outside fingers on the rim of the disc, two middle fingers underneath the disc, and your thumb should be placed underneath the disc near the center. Proper thumb placement ensures maximum stability. The four-finger grip is similar to the longhorn grip. The difference is that all your fingers are placed on the outside rim of the disc. With both grips you want to make sure the rim

of the disc is resting on the center point of your fingertips.

The turbo putt stance resembles one used to throw a baseball or softball (contralateral). For right-handers, place your left foot forward and right foot behind it (about shoulder width apart), and align your left leg so it is pointing directly at the target. You may also choose to use a staggered stance. Arm and wrist movements are critical to properly execute the turbo putt. Place your throwing arm to the side of your body and create a perpendicular angle with

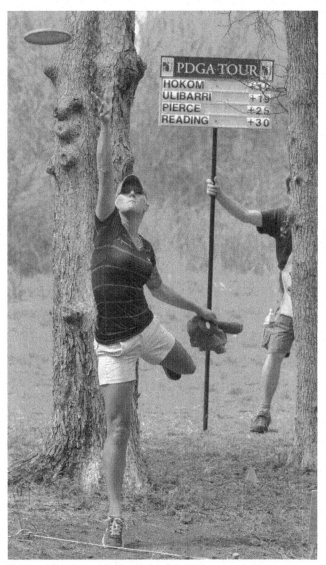

Catrina Allen drops a loft putt out of the sky. *Photo courtesy of PDGA Media*

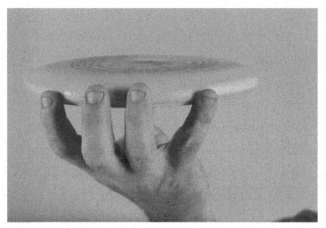

Turbo putt grips. *Photos by Ryan Bumgarner*

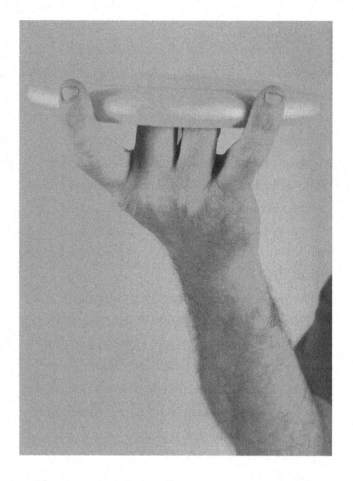

your arm so the disc is lying flat on your hand, utilizing one of the two recommended grips. Create a backward *L* shape with your upper arm and forearm so the disc rests in your hand at shoulder level or higher. Once your body and arm are in place, there is not a lot of arm movement needed to execute the putt. Shift your center of mass away from the target. Rotate your shoulders away from the target, and move your throwing arm back toward you. Keep your upper arm steady and pronate your wrist slightly. As you move your center of mass toward the target, rotate your shoulders and supinate your wrist. This action will create spin on the disc. On release, the front portion of the rim of the disc should be higher than the back rim (pitched up) unless faced with a strong tailwind or headwind.

Flick Putt

The **flick putt** is a forehand style of putt that uses mainly the wrist for execution. In reality, it is the same throw as the forehand **approach throw** with less arm action. When executing the flick putt, keep you forearm fairly still, and predominantly use wrist pop on release to accelerate the disc.

The best grip for the flick putt is the one that provides the most stability, which more times than not is the split finger grip described in chapter 9, on page 117. Since you do not need a lot of momentum on this putt, the index finger is best placed toward the center of the disc. Upon release, it is important to keep in mind the imaginary gun technique. The main movement of your hand mimics holding a gun, pointing it behind you and slightly toward the sky, and then bringing it to the target line at the release point. Make sure the front portion of the rim of the disc is pointing upward slightly. This will help the disc take an appropriate flight line to the target. It also helps ensure that the disc does not fly toward the ground on an anhyzer angle, which often results in bad roll-aways.

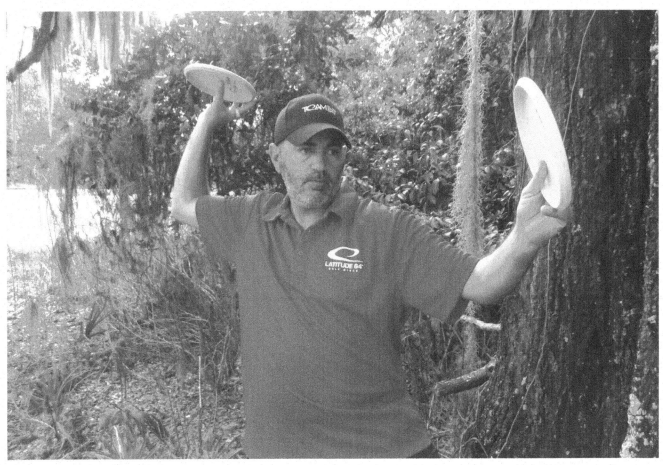

JohnE McCray's famous turbo putting form. *Photo by Jennifer McCray*

Jump Putt

The jump putt is a misnomer because according to the PDGA rule book it is not technically a putt. Jump putting inside 33 feet is against the rules, because your feet end up landing in front of your lie. As the name suggests, when executing a jump putt, a player literally jumps toward the target to create momentum. To execute a jump putt, shift your weight back slightly in your stance first, and then forward as you jump toward the target. Most players prefer an in-line stance and a spin style; however, a jump putt on a loft putt flight line can be a safe layup throw. For some players, this jump looks more like a slight leap, while others will execute a long, dynamic jump. The key to executing a successful jump putt is timing your arm extension with your peak jump height. If you think of a jump shooter in basketball timing his or her ball release with the apex of the jump, then you have the right idea. Because the jump requires more timing than other putts, your chances of making an error is increased.

Putting Tips

Regardless of the putting stance and style you choose to adopt, we offer the following five important putting tips. After reading this chapter in its entirety, we suggest referring to these tips often to help ensure your putting success.

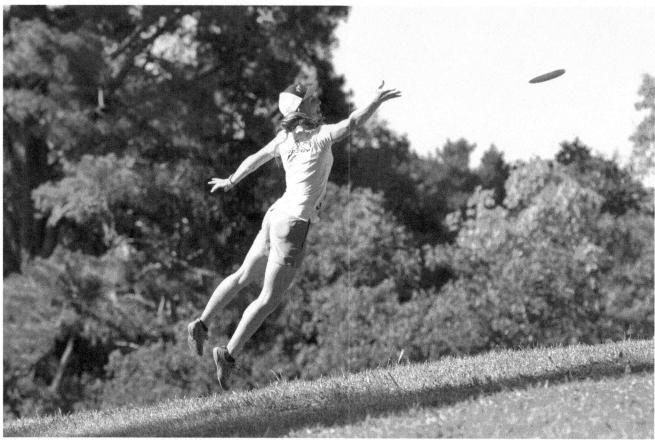

Paige Pierce's explosive jump-putting form. *Photo courtesy of PDGA Media*

Tip #1: Align Your Body

Make sure your body is in the proper position, starting from the ground up. If you are using an in-line stance, make sure your lead foot is lined up with the pole of the target and your back foot is on the same line. The majority of your weight should be on your lead foot (if using an in-line stance), with your lead leg slightly bent and stable. Find your center of balance (closing your eyes can help). Strive for a stance that feels stable, balanced, and comfortable.

Once you have your feet aligned with the pole, make sure your shoulders are level with the target. Some people like to point their throwing shoulder at the target while using an in-line stance, while others prefer to have both shoulders square (perpendicular) to the target. When using a straddle stance, align your shoulders square to the target. Either way, you will have more success if your shoulders are roughly level.

Tip #2: Aim with Your Thumb

Use your thumb to aim the disc and ensure it is on the proper flight line toward the target. If you look down your hand after release, your thumb and fingers should be lined up with the target. You can think of your thumb as an actual sight guide, similar to shooting a gun. Make sure that as you release the disc, your thumb is pointed at the middle of the target.

Tip #3: Use Your Legs

Extend (or "push") your rear leg when using an in-line stance or with both legs when using a straddle or staggered stance to move your center of balance toward the target. The amount of push is dependent on both the distance to the target and the style of putt. This push will likely cause your rear leg to lift off the ground slightly when using an in-line stance. When using a straddle or staggered stance, you may come up on your toes. Your spine should remain straight and you should avoid bending too much at the waist. When attempting shorter putts, you only have to move your center of balance an inch or so. You should avoid releasing the disc when your weight is over your back foot, unless you are faced with a difficult uphill lie on the fairway. Think of the push as a short, firm movement and not a forward lean.

Tip #4: Extend Toward the Target

Upon release, make sure that your arm is extended toward the chains of the target. Utilizing a wrist pop and an open-hand release will help ensure that the disc hits the chains. The quicker you extend your wrist, the more acceleration you gain on your putt. After you have released the disc, keep your hand open to help ensure proper follow-through. Think about your hand "greeting" the target as you extend your arm. The disc should feel as though it released cleanly out of your hand.

Tip #5: Focus on Disc Flight

When the positioning of your feet, arms, shoulders, and back come naturally, we recommend you focus on the flight of the disc. Imagine the disc leaving your hand, flying toward the target, and hitting the center of the chains. Occasionally ask a friend, teacher, or coach to evaluate your form. It is wise to focus on your form periodically, particularly when you are practicing the fundamentals. During competitive rounds, get your body in position and visualize the disc flying perfectly and banging the chains.

Analyzing the Green

Once you learn the fundamentals, the key to successful putting boils down to knowing the environmental variables that surround the target. It is important to analyze the green before you execute a putt by looking for obstacles, elevation changes, and low-hanging limbs. Better green analysis leads to fewer mistakes, which results in lower scores. Disc golf greens often have a variety of challenges and obstacles. Typically, they include elevation changes, trees, bushes, low-hanging limbs, and water.

Gauging where you are going to release the disc in relation to the elevation of the green will greatly improve your results. Analyzing green elevation is important because if you are putting uphill or downhill, you will need to adjust whether you release the disc above or slightly below your waist. The greater the elevation change, the more you will either want to release high or low. Another way to think about this is, using your throwing hand thumb as a guide, aim above the target for an uphill putt, and equal to or slightly below the target for a downhill putt. When putting uphill or downhill, maintain your balance, weight transfer, and extension the same as you would for a level green. Try adjusting only your aim.

The other variable you always want to keep in mind is the magnitude and direction of the wind.

You need to gauge if it is a headwind, tailwind, or a crosswind (and the direction of the crosswind). Wind direction is very important to understand; it informs you about how to position the lip or rim of the disc upon release. The wind affects the disc differently depending on the style of putt you use. Regardless of your style, make sure you are gauging wind direction and wind speed (more on wind in chapter 13).

Some players prefer to use the same putting stance and style no matter what environmental variables are present, including the wind. No matter what the situation is, they are going to putt exactly the same way every time. Still, there are other players who believe it is important to be able to execute several different types of putting styles depending on the situation. They would contest that, with this putting variability, they are able to switch putting styles to adjust to varying conditions.

Spin putts are excellent any time when you have a long putt, about 30 to 120 feet from the target. During heavy winds is also an excellent time to use the spin putt, especially if you are challenged with headwinds or crosswinds. Since the flight of the disc is on a relatively straight line to the target, it has less time in the air; hence the wind will affect it less. A spin putt on a slight anhyzer line is also a wise choice for uphill greens. The extra momentum created with a spin putt will help compensate for the uphill elevation change, and you will have less chance of leaving your putt short.

If faced with a downhill putt, a spin putt might not be a wise choice, as it can leave you with an extremely long comeback putt. Of course, you do not want to be thinking about the dreaded triple putt before you release the disc. When you perform a putt, you want your mind to be clear. The last thing you want to be thinking is, *Wow, if I miss this putt I might be 50 feet away with a second putt coming back.* If this is the case, you might be better off switching to a different putting style.

Another situation when a spin putt is not an ideal choice is when you are challenged with a strong tailwind. Oftentimes a tailwind will cause a disc to quickly lose loft, and you will end up short of the target. This, of course, depends on your putting technique and the angle of the disc upon release. A lot of players who use spin putts will keep the front portion of the rim up and the back part down (pitched up) on release. If this is your preferred technique, you should realize it will need to be changed with a tailwind, or you will need to aim a lot higher than normal. A tailwind will drive the disc down, and you will likely miss low.

Loft putts are excellent to use when you have extremely steep greens or drop-offs behind the target. When using a loft putt, you do not have to worry about missing the target and then facing a dreaded 45- to 50-foot comeback putt. If you miss the target when executing a loft putt, your disc will often come to rest about 15 feet from the target because of the sharp downward flight of the disc.

The loft putt is also a wise choice if the green has low-lying bushes between you and the target, blocking a straight flight plane. In this situation, a spin putt may be difficult to execute. The upward and downward flight pattern of the loft putt allows the disc to elevate loft upon release, fly over the bushes, and then down near the target as it loses loft. We have witnessed push putts elevate as high as 12 feet over a small bush to then land in the target after traveling nearly 35 feet.

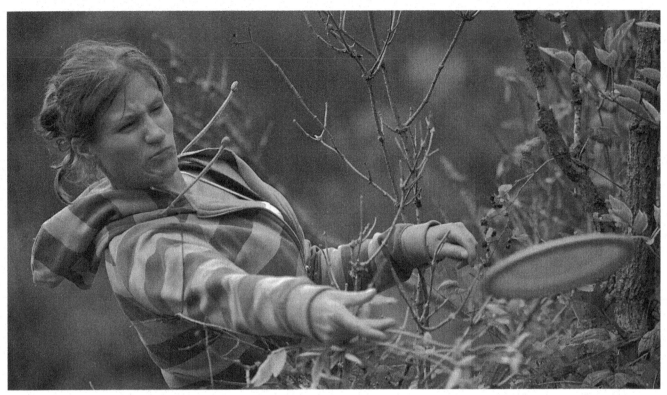

Maria Smirnovskaya flick-putts her way out of trouble. *Photo by Martin Frederiksen*

A scenario in which it makes sense to execute a turbo put is when you have a drastic elevation change directly under your putting stance and one of your legs is several feet lower than the other. This position makes it extremely tough to get your shoulders square to the target, which means you must compensate for the change in the release by switching putting styles. In this scenario, the turbo putt allows you to release the disc in a flat position and in-line with the target.

If your lie is behind a tree or bush, or you need to get a better angle to the target due to some other obstacle, a flick putt might be a wise choice. It is very easy to straddle while using this putt, which allows you to stretch your body around obstacles to access the greater percentage of open space and a more advantageous flight line. Some players will switch to a flick putt when they are faced with an uphill putt that is out of their normal putting style range.

Flick putts can be dangerous if you have steep angles or immediate drop-offs around the green. The release angles of most flick putts can cause a roll-away, especially when the target is placed on a steep slope. The optimal throwing angle can be either an anhyzer or hyzer depending on the obstacle you are trying to putt around. If you face a challenging drop-off, a missed flick putt may fly even farther away from the target, and you will be left with a long comeback putt.

Jump putts are only used on longer putts. We do not recommend jump-putting if you are inside about 40 feet. When you are jumping, you create more movement with your body, which creates error-producing variables. If you practice executing long spin putts, you will find you can execute putts from about 80 feet without having to use a jump putt. However, if you are already highly skilled at jump-putting, we do not suggest you stop using this technique. Still, it is important for novice players to develop putting techniques that minimize potentially error-producing variables, and jump-putting demands additional timing and greater opportunity for error.

Practice Techniques to Improve Your Putting

Of course, one of the keys to putting practice is to do it often, daily if possible. The easiest way to make this happen is to set up a target in your backyard or local practice area. There are many different targets available for about $150. If you do not have the money to purchase a target, you can easily use a wooden stake, PVC pipe, or fence post. In actuality, hitting a post or a stake is much more difficult than hitting the chains of a target. So if you practice putting at a post or stake and learn to hit it consistently, then your putting percentage may improve on an official target.

Some people prefer to putt with a disc or towel in their non-throwing hand. If you prefer this technique during competitive rounds, we recommend you do it when practicing. One common mistake is holding several discs in your non-throwing hand while practicing. If you prefer to have an empty non-throwing hand during competitive rounds, pick each putter off the ground one at a time when you practice.

We recommend you practice putting at least 20 minutes each day. Taking 50 to 100 practice putts on a regular basis can improve your game significantly over a period of one year or less. We recommend acquiring 5 to 10 of the same make and model of putters to use during practice. Ideally, you should use the same makes and models for practicing as you use in competition. If you are a novice player, purchasing a few different putters is fine until you find one or two you like. We typically carry two or more different putters in our tournament bags, a go-to putter and a disc that is a bit overstable, to use in the wind or for approach throws.

When you practice putting, do not try to make long putts until you are fairly consistently hitting short-range putts. Oftentimes players will attempt very long putts instead of working on the essential 20- to 30-foot range. We recommend you start with short-range putts and track your percentages, meaning keep track of how well you do at various distances. Stay at that distance until you are at least 50 percent successful. The best putters in the world make about 90 percent of their putts inside 30 feet. Outside 30 feet, the best players are about 60 percent successful.

One great technique we have learned to track distance is creating distance markers on your backyard putting green. This can be very easily accomplished by placing bricks in the ground at different distances from the target or by using marker paint. We recommend you start with 15-foot putts and increase your distance by increments of five feet. Perform 6 to 10 putts at each distance. Do not move farther away from the target until you make at least 50 percent of your putts. Some folks like to keep a written logbook of putting percentages, and we think that is a great idea.

Move the target around your yard or practice area to practice elevated putts. Practice putting from difficult stances (e.g., on a slope or wet surface). Also, practicing in the wind and adverse weather conditions will greatly improve your putting when the weather turns foul. In this way, you will learn to be comfortable in these conditions and will know how to throw a wet disc. Practice putting around and over bushes, trees, signs, etc. Perhaps you have heard the saying "Practice makes perfect." Well, there is no scientific evidence that is true. In reality, variable practice makes you better in varied conditions.

When practicing putting, it is very important to treat each putt as if you were playing in a competitive round of golf. We see a lot of people putting with many different types of discs (even drivers). Oftentimes, they quickly throw at the target as if they are a putting machine gun with rapid-fire action. This is a very poor practice strategy. There are better ways to warm up your arm without developing bad habits. Instead, practice each and every putt by getting set and going through all the steps of your normal routine. In other words, attempt each putt as you would during an actual round of play. Take your time and develop a consistent routine that allows you to quickly get comfortable.

Keep your pre-putting routine to 10 or 15 seconds before you release the disc. If you look at the top putters in the game, they might have a couple quirks or interesting movements during their putting routine, but by and large their putting routine is pretty much the same each time. It is always the same process, and it tends to be pretty quick and simple. Your putting routine should include the following:

1. Check for elevation changes, wind direction, and obstacles.
2. Align feet and body with the target.
3. Check that you have a legal foot placement.
4. Find your center of balance.
5. Aim at one chain link on the target.
6. Imagine the disc flying through the air and hitting the chains.

On a challenging course, it is likely you will use each of these putting styles at some point during a round. So you might as well get comfortable using all the different styles of putts. At least one day a week, incorporate practice for each of the different putting styles and stances. Of course, if you are tracking your results, make sure you identify the style of putt used on that day.

Some players like to play games when they practice putting. Games like **Hott Shott**, **Around the World**, and **Ring of Fire** are fun ways to compete with your friends. However, we believe quality putting practice is best done by yourself. After all, when you are standing over your marker before an important putt during a competitive round, it is only your thoughts and behaviors that matter. You may never be physically able to drive 450 feet, but anyone can become a better putter with quality skill practice and the desire to improve.

Chapter 13

Before Every Throw

When you are out enjoying a round of disc golf, there are four important variables you should scrutinize before you decide which disc to retrieve from your bag, which type of throw to execute, and which throwing angle to use. These variables often change substantially with every throw you attempt on the course. Understanding how to recognize these variables and plan accordingly is critical to the success of each throw. This constant and sometimes pressure-filled strategizing is part of what makes disc golf both a challenging and addicting sport. These internal planning sessions can be rewarding when you get it right and frustrating when you do not. Regardless of the course you are playing or the type of round (casual, practice, or competitive), disc selection and throw execution should be based on the following variables:

1. Footing/stance
2. Percentage of open space
3. Elevation changes and slant
4. Wind direction and intensity

Analyze Your Footing/Stance

Look at the ground (or tee pad) beneath your feet. Is there anything that could potentially affect your stance such as tree roots, rocks, loose gravel, grass, leaves, weeds, mud, wood chips, or snow? Can you throw from a level stance, or are you faced with an uphill or downhill stance? Is the surface slippery? Can you use an X-step or two-step approach (explained in the next chapter), or should you throw from a standstill? It may sound like a lot to ask, which is why you should begin planning for your next throw before you reach your lie. After you stand behind your mini marker, you only have about 30 seconds or so to think about these variables. So start planning before you reach your lie.

The key concept is to play the hand you have been dealt. Both X-steps and two-steps can create a lot of momentum, but if you do not have the room or the proper footing to execute them, you may be better off throwing from a standstill. Experienced players know that if the surface is slippery or treacherous, executing an X-step or two-step can lead to disastrous results. When in doubt, stand and throw.

If your lie is on a severe slant (from left to right or right to left as you face the target), it may be difficult to keep your shoulders level with the ground. In these circumstances, consider throwing an overhand or forehand throw. If faced with a downhill stance (your lead foot is lower than your back foot), consider using an anhyzer throwing angle (either forehand or backhand). If you have an uphill stance (your lead foot is higher than your back foot), consider using an anhyzer throwing angle (either forehand or backhand). It is a lot to consider, but take a deep breath—30 seconds is ample time to contemplate your throwing style and throwing angle options.

Inexperienced players often use their go-to throwing style on every throw, even if the lie (and ultimately the stance) calls for something else. Remember, subtle tweaks to your stance can lead to very different flight patterns. On densely wooded courses with significant elevation changes, you may be lucky to have 18 throws from a dry, level stance that is free of impediments. At times, you may even have to throw (putt, in particular) from your knees. Incorporating different stances in your practice routine is helpful, but nothing beats playing rounds on a variety of courses when it comes to improving your ability to throw from various stances with success.

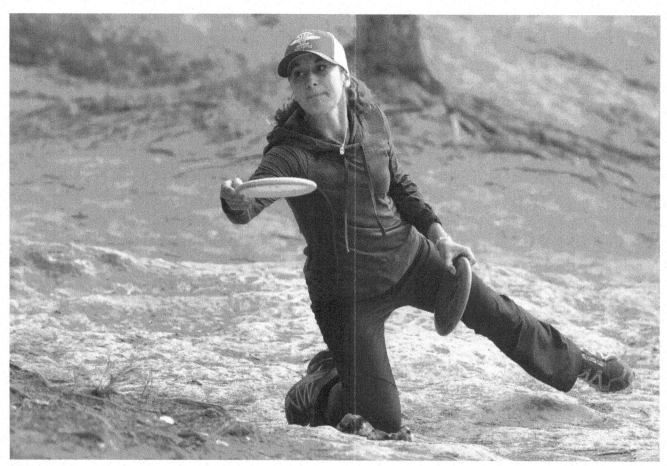

Jessica Weese opts for a kneeling stance. *Photo courtesy of PDGA Media*

Identify the Greatest Percentage of Open Space

The next important variable you need to consider before every throw is the percentage of open space. The percentage of open space is the amount of airspace available for each potential flight path or route. From the tee pad (or on the second or third throw on a par-4 or par-5), there may be several routes to the target or landing area. The key is to examine all the possible routes and assess the percentage of open space for each route. On wide-open holes, the open space is everywhere. When you are scrambling on tightly wooded courses, open space may be hard to find.

The principle of the greatest percentage of open space works simply. If you have a route that has absolutely no obstructions (i.e., no trees, hanging vines, telephone poles, electrical wires, or other possible disc deflectors), then you have a route with 100 percent open space. If a route has several large trees, you may estimate they are taking up about 20 percent of the route, therefore leaving you with roughly 80 percent of open space. Again, the important concept here is to take what the course gives you. More often than not, you should choose the route with the greatest percentage of open space, which thus affords the greatest chance of success. Some throws tempt you with two routes each with roughly 50 percent open space. In these

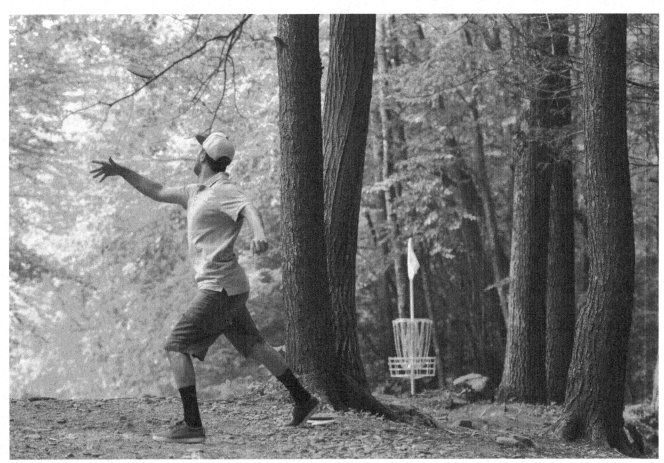

Taylor Maz just misses a low-hanging branch protecting the green on hole 7 at the Maple Hill Gold disc golf course in Leicester, Massachusetts. *Photo courtesy of PDGA Media*

situations, go with your best throwing style (e.g., a backhand or forehand).

To capitalize on the greatest percentage of open space, you must be versatile. Beginners will often use their go-to throwing style on every throw, even if the percentage of open space calls for something else. To become an advanced or professional player, you need the ability to execute most of the various throwing styles described in pervious chapters with consistency. These throws include the backhand, forehand, thumber, tomahawk, and roller from various throwing angles (from a steep hyzer to a steep anhyzer). You do not have to be adept at all these throws to play well, but developing a good bit of versatility will greatly improve your scores.

Account for Elevation Changes and Slant

Elevation changes are deviations in the height of the fairway from the tee pad to the green or landing area. Of course, throwing steeply uphill or downhill is a common challenge on many disc golf holes. Accounting for elevation changes before every throw will undoubtedly elicit greater success. As we mentioned previously, using a forehand or overhand throwing style is often a wise choice when faced with severe elevation changes.

Throwing downhill can lead to greater distance, if you get the pitch angle correct. The most common mistake is releasing the disc at an angle that is parallel to the tee pad (or ground beneath your feet) instead of parallel to the downward angle of the fairway. Remember, your shoulders (and ultimately the disc, on release) should be roughly level with the ground, which is fairly easy to do when the fairway is level (zero elevation gain or loss). If you are throwing a backhand downhill, your shoulders (and the disc, on release) should be

about level with the angle of the fairway. If you are throwing from a level tee pad, your throwing shoulder should be below your non-throwing one, and the disc should be released at a downward pitch angle or "nose down" a bit. A disc thrown level with the tee pad on a downhill fairway will often result in a flight pattern that is too steep/high. Discs thrown too high downhill are often doomed from the start.

An important concept to remember is that discs thrown downhill have a tendency to fade and glide more than discs thrown on a level flight line. If you are trying to throw straight downhill, consider using a disc that is more understable than you would use normally. If you have the open space, downhill turnover and S-shots seem to glide forever. If you need to shape your throw and you have the distance to reach the green or landing area, using a hyzer throwing angle can yield great results. The idea is that if you know the disc is going to fade significantly anyway, use an overstable disc on a steep hyzer line and plan on it fading like crazy.

Although it may not appear so to a novice player, throwing uphill is markedly easier than throwing downhill. Sure, it is challenging to throw a great distance uphill, but uphill throwing errors seem to be less penalizing than downhill ones. The most common mistake is not releasing the disc nose-up a bit, often resulting in a woefully short throw. If you are using a backhand throwing style, your throwing shoulder should be above your non-throwing one slightly, and you should release the disc at an upward pitch angle or "nose up" a bit. Consider using a disc that is more overstable than you would normally use if you have space for an S-shot. Backhand throws that slowly turn over can work quite well when faced with an uphill throw, if thrown roughly flat. Use caution when

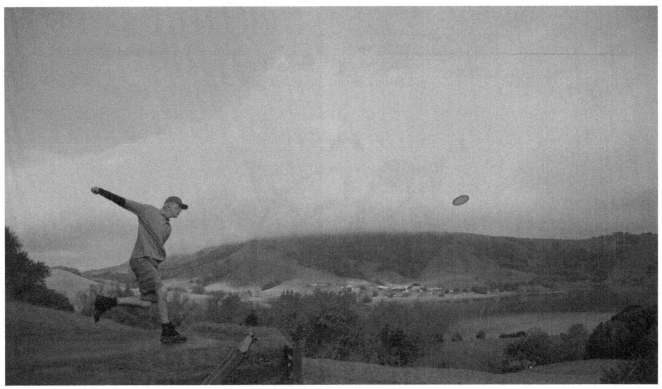

Bill Sherman bombs a downhill drive at Stafford Lake County Park in Novato, California. *Photo by Martin Frederiksen*

attempting a hyzer throwing angle uphill. When in doubt, throw a forehand unless an overhead throw is more your style. Before you take elevation into account, consider the percentage of open space. The more open space, the more throwing style options available.

In addition to accounting for elevation changes of the fairway, it is important to scrutinize the slant of the green or landing area. Some greens or landing areas are flat, but others slant (also called slope) from left to right or right to left. Keep in mind that backhands will often hit the ground at an angle that mirrors those of forehands. In other words, a backhand hyzer will hit the ground at an angle that is the opposite of a forehand hyzer, but they both will be spinning clockwise. As a result, two different throws that hit the ground in the exact same spot can come to rest in vastly different places. When hyzers hit the ground, they tend to keep spinning (or end up rolling), while anhyzers tend to land a bit more flat. As discussed earlier, overhead throws can bounce or land upside down and slide. There are so many potential combinations (e.g., a forehand hyzer thrown right-handed to a left-to-right-sloping green will tend to slide away from where it hits the ground) that it seems pointless to try and list them all. As we discussed in previous chapters, the only way to learn is to implement practice variability, including landing discs on various slopes.

Gauge the Wind Direction and Intensity

The wind direction and intensity can have a significant effect on the lift, glide, and stability of a thrown disc, hence gauging the wind before every throw is essential. Are you facing a headwind, tailwind, or crosswind? If it is a crosswind, which

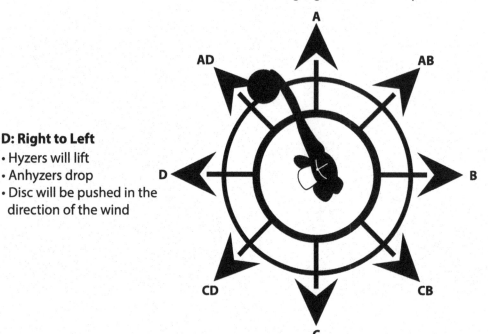

A: Downwind (Tailwind)
- More carry
- Drops faster
- Discs become more overstable
- Low angle ground effect skips

D: Right to Left
- Hyzers will lift
- Anhyzers drop
- Disc will be pushed in the direction of the wind

B: Left to Right
- Hyzers will drop
- Anhyzers will lift
- Disc will be pushed in the direction of the wind

C: Upwind (Headwind)
- Must force carry
- Disc rises
- Shorter, more vertical skips
- Disc become less stable

Wind compass. *Original illustration courtesy of Discraft and recreated by Scott Clontz*

direction is the wind blowing? To help answer these questions, try tossing a few blades of grass, some leaves, or a bit of dirt into the air before your throw; just make sure whatever you toss does not blow on the other players in your group.

Ron Convers Jr. and Brendan Hickman wrote an excellent article titled "Mastering the Wind." We like their sage advice on disc selection when throwing in the wind: If you choose an overstable disc in wind conditions, you will only be right about half the time. Disc selection is important

when throwing in windy conditions, but you must first evaluate the wind's direction and intensity.

Tailwinds have the potential to add distance to your throw, especially if you throw using a forehand style. Tailwinds will also tend to push a disc down toward the ground; therefore it is imperative that you use a slightly higher release point to compensate for this effect. This is especially true when putting with an intense tailwind. It is not unusual to witness putts dropping several feet in intense tailwinds. Using a disc at the understable end of the continuum when faced with a tailwind is typically a good idea.

Headwinds tend to lift a disc higher up in the air and lessen its stability, meaning the disc will likely turn or flip faster than normal. The keys to throwing in a headwind are to make sure you aim lower than normal and to release the disc at a downward pitch angle (called nose down). If you release the disc at an upward pitch angle, you will witness the power of a headwind as it gets under the rim of the disc and pushes it high in the air. Using a disc toward the overstable end of the continuum is generally a good idea when faced with intense headwinds.

Right-to-left crosswinds will push a right-handed backhand (RHBH) thrown with an anhyzer throwing angle toward the ground and may even cause an unintentional roller. Discs thrown at an anhyzer throwing angle may lift and glide more than expected. Overstable discs thrown relatively flat or less stable discs thrown at a slight hyzer angle tend to work well for right-to-left crosswinds. Imagine the release angle of the disc "knifing" or "fighting" the wind direction instead of "succumbing" to it. Typically, left-to-right crosswinds will push an RHBH hyzer toward the ground and anhyzers will be lifted up in the air.

Some of the most advantageous and most challenging winds are called **quarterwinds**. These occur when the wind is a combination of a headwind or tailwind and a crosswind. Picture yourself in the middle of a compass as illustrated on page 160. To use this guide, pick the direction your disc has to fly to avoid obstacles. Remember, as your disc flies, the wind will affect the disc differently depending on the throwing angle (hyzer, anhyzer, or flat) and the direction of flight.

Combine the directions on the chart for alternate winds (e.g. AB, AD, CB, etc.). If the direction is more *A* than *B*, the wind will be more *A* than *B*.

If faced with a tailwind that is blowing right to left, throwing an overstable disc at an anhyzer angle may afford a straighter and higher flight path (see the illustration on page 162). The anhyzer angle of the disc on release may prevent the crosswind from lifting it considerably. Because a less stable disc should be thrown at a hyzer angle, the crosswind will likely push it and cause it to lift. Because of the tailwind, you should choose a disc that is less stable than one you would normally use on a calm day.

When faced with a headwind that is also blowing right to left, a less stable disc should be thrown on a hyzer angle (see the illustration on page 163). A more stable disc on an anhyzer throwing angle will likely turn/flip/roll slightly and then fade sharply toward the end of flight. In either case, a disc thrown slightly lower than normal is optimal. When faced with this type of wind, consider choosing a disc that is slightly more overstable than you would normally choose on a calm day.

When challenged with a headwind that is also blowing left to right, avoid throwing at an anhyzer angle (see the illustration on page 164). Instead, consider throwing an overstable disc flat, or a less stable disc on a hyzer angle. This hyzer angle will likely cause the disc to drop considerably. If you do not choose a disc that is overstable enough, or it is not thrown at a steep enough hyzer angle, it will very likely turn/flip/roll and miss the green or landing area to the right.

If faced with a tailwind that is also blowing left to right, you can throw a less stable and slower disc

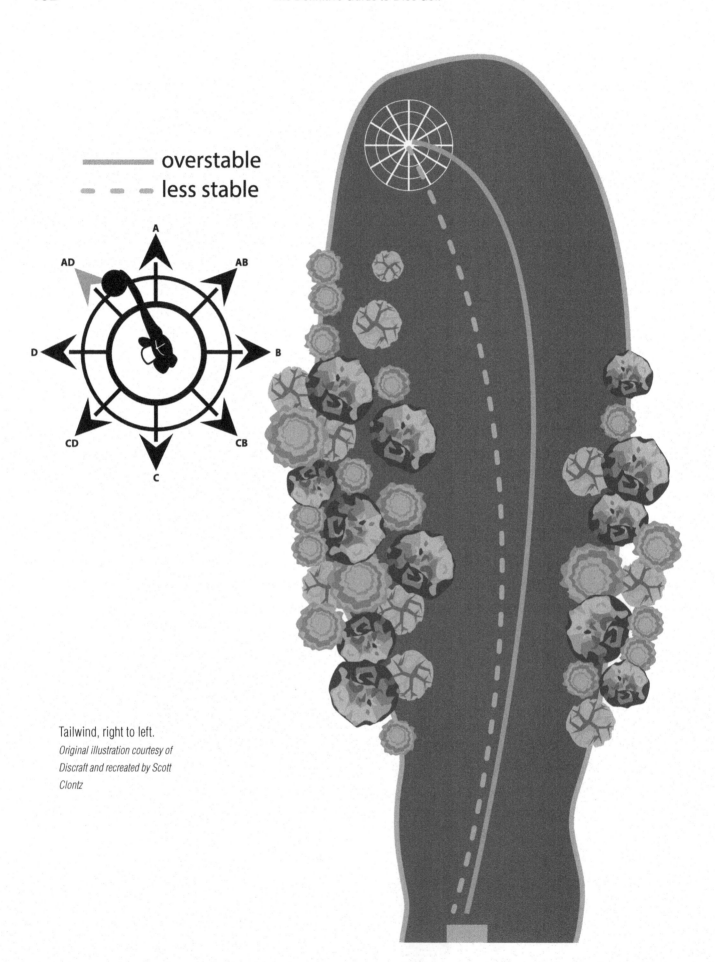

overstable

less stable

Tailwind, right to left.
Original illustration courtesy of
Discraft and recreated by Scott
Clontz

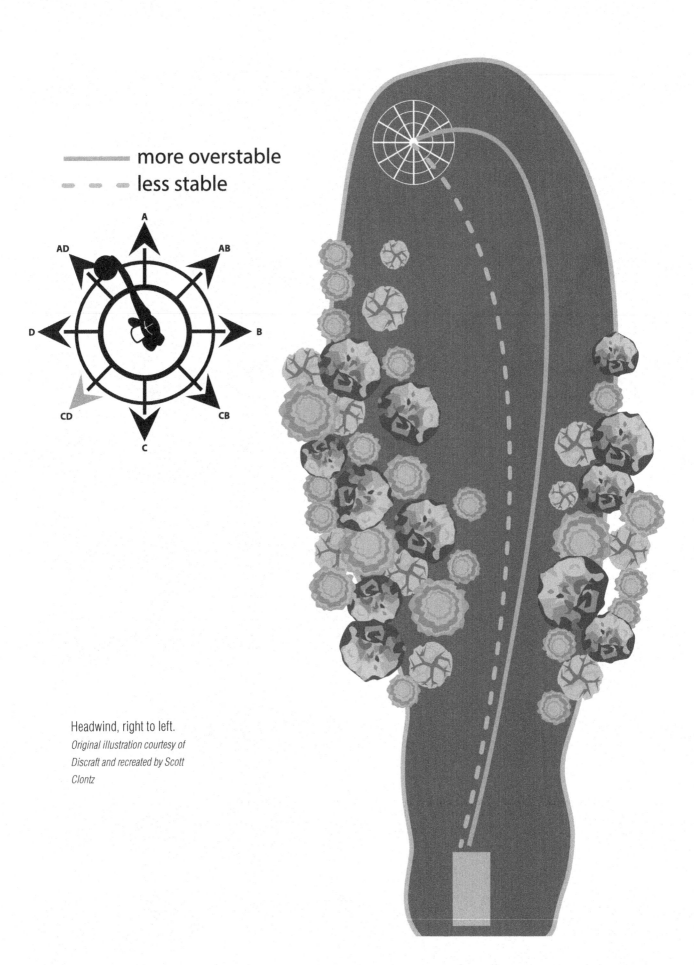

more overstable

less stable

Headwind, right to left.
Original illustration courtesy of Discraft and recreated by Scott Clontz

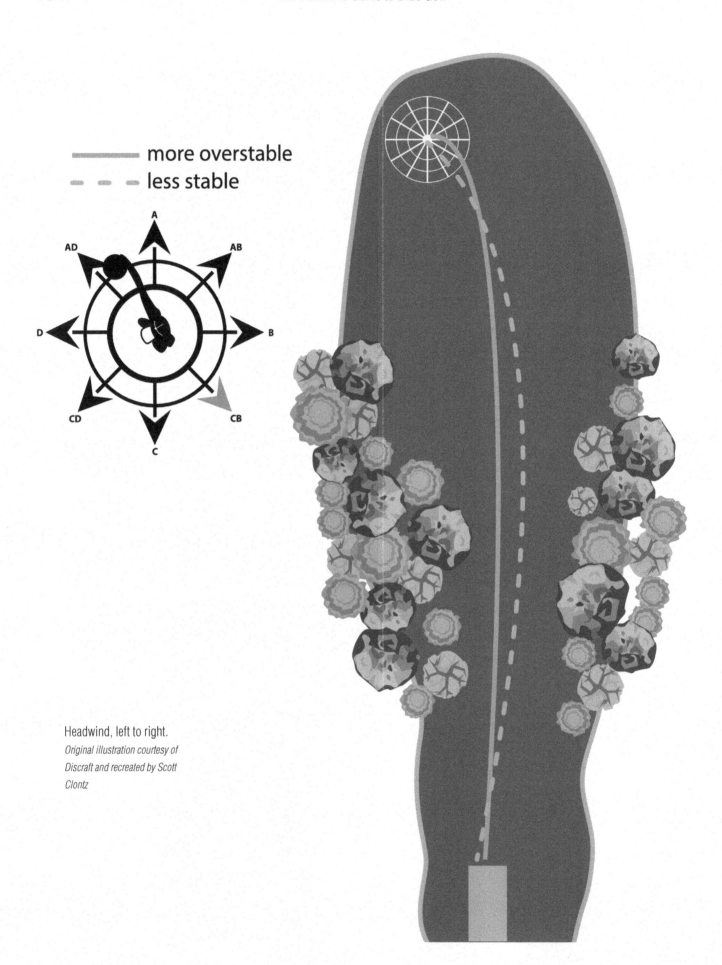

more overstable

less stable

Headwind, left to right.
Original illustration courtesy of Discraft and recreated by Scott Clontz

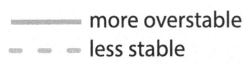

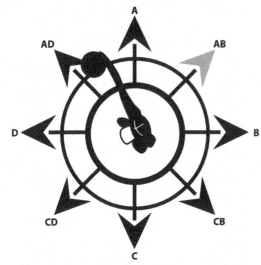

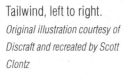

Tailwind, left to right.
Original illustration courtesy of Discraft and recreated by Scott Clontz

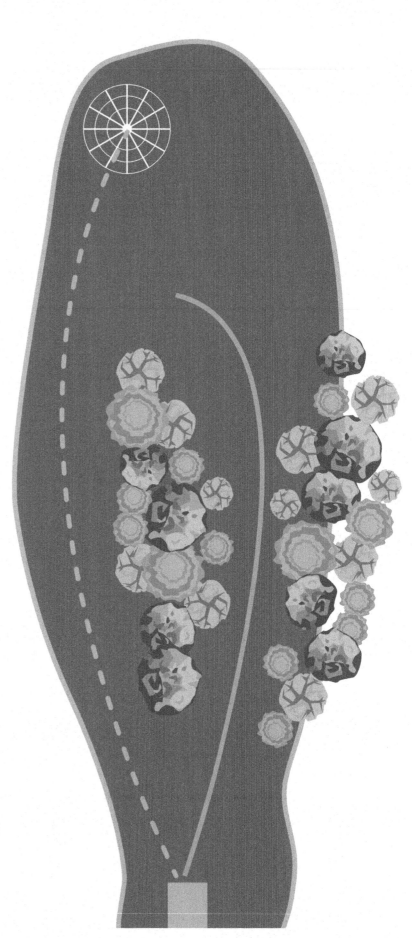

much farther than normal (see the illustration on page 165). The crosswind may create lift and will push the disc to the right. A more stable disc at a hyzer angle of release with this wind will likely cause it to drop quickly. Consider using a much less stable disc and throw it flat or at a slight hyzer angle. If you can throw an RHBH with significant velocity, it is fun to try a hyzer flip in this wind.

Before you decide on which disc to use, which style of throw to execute, and which throwing angle to attempt, it is wise to first analyze your stance, identify the greatest percentage of open space, account for elevation changes, and gauge the wind direction and intensity. Of course, there are many times when the stance, open space, elevation, and wind do not call for the same throw. When faced with this dilemma, you must decide which variable is most critical to success. There is no substitute for playing experience, but no matter how much you play, your stance may be challenging, the percentage of open space may be difficult to determine, elevation changes may seem problematic, and the wind may still fool you.

Chapter 14

Approach Throw Fundamentals

The best way to be successful at traditional golf is to learn to hit your short irons and wedges from the tee box, fairway grass, and rough well enough to consistently give yourself a chance at a birdie putt. In disc golf, your short irons and wedges are equivalent to your midrange and putt/approach discs. This chapter will outline the biomechanical movement patterns, practice conditions, and cognitive strategies essential for executing approach throws with success.

The objective of an approach throw (also called an upshot) is to land the disc as close to the target or desired landing area as possible. Successful approach throws result in easy "gimme" putts or lies on the fairway with a clear flight line to the target. Approach throws range from about 50 to 300 feet and can be executed using backhands, forehands, thumbers, tomahawks, or rollers. Most often, players will choose a midrange or putt/approach disc when executing an approach throw, although there are circumstances when a fairway driver or driver is an appropriate choice, even on shorter approach throws.

Biomechanics of Approach Throws

As mentioned, there are four variables you should consider before deciding which type and style of throw to use. If your footing for an upshot is relatively flat, without impediments, and you have room to move a bit, you may choose to use a two-step approach in lieu of an X-step. But remember, more movement means more potential for error, especially if you have a difficult stance. However, executing a two-step can help create rhythm, momentum, and greater torque than a standstill throw.

To execute a basic two-step approach, start with your body facing the target. If throwing a right-handed backhand (RHBH), your first movement is to take one small step with your left foot. Lift it up off the ground and then turn it to the left so, when placed on the ground, it is roughly perpendicular to the intended target. For shorter throws, you may barely step at all. Changing the position of your left foot will allow you to load your hips, rotate your spine, and turn your shoulders. Next, take a step toward your intended target with your right (lead) foot. While your leg is in the air, pivot your front foot so when it lands your heel is pointed

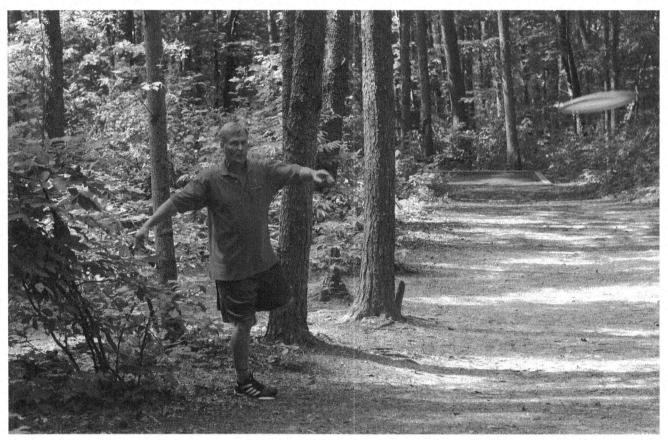

Eric "the Legend" Marx executes a backhand approach throw at Richmond Hill in Asheville, North Carolina. *Photo by Cyndy Caravelis*

toward the target and your toes are pointed 120° away from the target. Depending on the intended throwing angle, it should be about in line with your left (rear) foot. Your feet should now be in the same stance used for an RHBH standstill throw. Your body should be in the ideal position to reach back with your throwing arm. As you snap your hips and rotate your spine, your throwing arm should pull the disc close to your body then extend to the release point. After release, your right foot should pivot clockwise to help execute an appropriate follow-through. Many players choose to use a fan grip for approach throws, although longer throws may necessitate using a three-finger or power grip.

Two-step approaches for forehands and rollers follow the same fundamental movement pattern as described for RHBH throws. Of course, when

throwing a right-handed forehand (RHFH), you should begin the two-step approach with your right foot. Having a quick forehand two-step in your bag of tricks can be extremely valuable on the course, because you can keep your eyes on your target.

There is one variation worth mentioning that is more of a stationary setup. Forehands can be used from behind trees or other obstacles because you can "straddle out" from your lie by leaning into a wide sideways stance. In this way, you may take obstacles out of play and create a different angle to the intended target. Remember to check for a legal stance in these situations. When executing these forehand throws (also called flicks), there is very little body movement, as these throws are executed primarily with your throwing arm and wrist pop

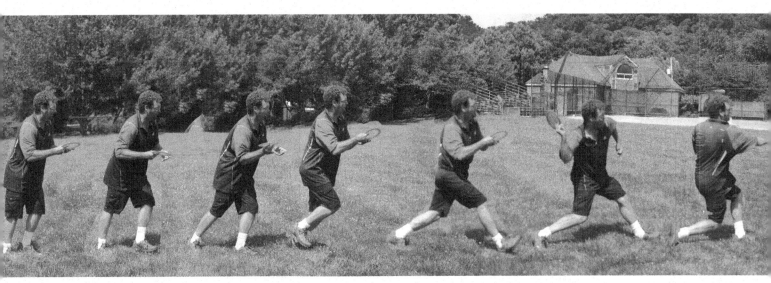

Ryan Pickens demonstrates a forehand two-step approach. *Photo by Cyndy Caravelis*

(or flick) on release. The grip typically used for this throw is the two-fingered forehand grip.

Practice Techniques for Improving Approach Throws

When executing approach throws (or driving from a tee pad on some par-3 holes), most players opt to use a midrange or a putt/approach disc, although using a fairway driver is not uncommon. You can choose to use a flat, hyzer, or anhyzer throwing angle using a backhand, forehand, thumber, tomahawk, or roller style of throw. Improving your ability to execute approach throws is critical to scoring well on modern courses, where it is common to see par-4 and par-5 holes that range from 350 to 600 feet. Throwing a disc 300 feet and landing it cleanly on the fairway is impressive, but if you cannot land your next throw close to the intended target or landing area, your beautiful drive may feel like a wasted throw.

We recommend several different methods for practicing your short game. Ideally, you should own about five midrange discs of the same make, model,

and weight to optimize practice time. Of course, this may not be a feasible expectation for many novice players. Some players prefer to use about five slightly different versions (of varying types of plastic) of the same make and model of midrange disc. In addition, many advanced and professional players will use several discs of the same make, model, weight, *and plastic type* that are in various stages of "beatness." Remember, seasoned or "beat in" discs tend to turn more and fade less.

As we discussed in chapters 8 through 11, practicing different throws (e.g., backhand on a hyzer throwing angle) about five to seven times in succession is an effective practice technique. Once you learn the fundamentals of each type of throw, you can take advantage of a **contextual interference** effect. Normally interference seems like a bad thing, but in this case it is not.

It works like this: When you execute the same throw in succession (ideally using the same make, model, and weight of disc), you are able to observe the same basic flight pattern from one throw to the next. You can also make subtle but important changes to your movement patterns and analyze how those changes affect the next throw. Of course, this is valuable practice time. When you switch to a different throw after five to seven trials (e.g., from a backhand hyzer to an anhyzer), you stay cognitively engaged in the process and may find that you ask and attempt to answer important questions like "How does an anhyzer *fly* differently from a hyzer?" or "How does throwing an anhyzer *feel* different from throwing a hyzer?" When executing too many of the same throw in succession, our experience and research indicates that learners tend to "put their minds on autopilot," mindlessly throwing the same type of throw over and over again. Mixing it up ultimately leads to much better long-term results from practice. Remember, it is not about developing "muscle memory." Quality practice requires both cognitive and physical engagement.

In a perfect world, all your midrange throws (either from the tee pad or fairway) will come to rest within 25 feet of the target. Some call this 25-foot radius around the target the **circle of love**. If you aspire to be a professional, you should strive to land about 80 percent of your midrange throws in the circle of love. Of course, the closer you are to the target to begin with, the more likely you are to land in the circle. If your disc comes to rest in the circle of love after a drive from the tee pad, your playing partners may let out an audible "Parked." If you want to park your approach throws and short drives from the tee pad, you should practice your throws and not simply play competitive rounds.

When practicing midrange throws, it is a good idea to develop a way to track your percentages. In this way, you will know which types of throws need the most improvement. First, get a measuring tape and field paint and draw a 25-foot circle around your portable target. If you do not have

field paint, flour works quite well, although it will not last as long. Next, mark spots on the ground approximately 100, 150, 200, and 250 feet from the target. Practice your throws as suggested, and track the percentage of your throws that come to rest in the circle of love. Practice on a flat field or other outdoor space to establish a baseline measure of distance before attempting uphill or downhill approaches. If you are a beginner, there is no reason to practice throwing from 150 and 200 feet if you are not already landing at least 50 percent of your discs in the circle. Instead, mark spots from 50, 75, and 100 feet. Once you are consistently landing 50 percent or more of your discs in the circle, then begin to throw from 150 to 200 feet.

Midrange throws can be practiced anywhere, but using a wide-open field is ideal. When you throw in a field, you can really get a sense for how the discs are flying without any obstructions or variables other than wind. If you choose to practice on a football or soccer field, it should be relatively easy to figure out where 100, 150, and 200 feet are, because these fields will have marked lines. The other advantage of throwing on athletic fields is that they often have goal posts. Throwing between the goal posts is an excellent way to develop throwing precision. When playing great courses, you will be challenged to throw through small gaps between trees as narrow as eight feet, and 20-foot gaps are fairly common. Fortunately, football goal posts are just wider than 18 feet wide. Position yourself about 100 feet away from the goal posts and throw five to seven forehands, backhands, and overhands through the gap. Once you are able to get 80 percent of your throws through the goal posts, move back to 150, 200, and 250 feet and track your percentages. Again, your goal should be a success rate of 80 percent or better if you aspire to play professionally.

You can also practice throwing anhyzers and hyzers through the goal posts. Instead of standing straight in front of the goal posts, move to the right or to the left by about 50 to 80 feet and practice hyzers and anhyzers by attempting to fly the disc between the posts. This can be an extremely effective way to practice. Once you begin to master hyzers and anhyzers from 100 feet, challenge yourself by again moving back to 125, 150, 200, and 250 feet until you are able to achieve an 80 percent success rate there. If you achieve this, you are ready to be a disc golf professional, assuming you are a phenomenal putter and can drive a disc about 400 feet.

Another excellent way to practice your midrange game is to create a short course around your home or neighborhood. If you do not have the money to purchase several targets, **object courses** can easily be laid out by placing tall stakes, PVC posts, or fence posts in the ground. If you do not want to go to that extent, just map out a course with already established targets like trees, sign posts, or fire hydrants. Having an object course in your backyard or neighborhood can be an excellent way to get out for 30 minutes or so and practice your game. Instead of keeping score, take five to seven discs and throw them all at each target. Of course, you can also track how many of them you park on each hole.

Ideally, you want to design your home course in a way that challenges you to practice different throws. For example, hole 1 could afford you the opportunity to practice a backhand anhyzer. Hole 2 could be a straight throw, but hole 3

might beg for a forehand hyzer. Your home course could emphasize approach throws by keeping the distances of the holes to 250 feet or less. As you play the course, you have the opportunity to practice all the different midrange throws to improve your game. If you do not have the room to set up a course in your backyard (or your neighbors are not happy when you throw discs from the street), then we recommend you visit a local park to create a course or find the local recreational disc golf course in your area. Not everyone has the space to create a home course, and parking your DX Roc on your neighbor's barbecue grill is never a good idea. In this case, you are better off heading to your local recreational course.

Recreational courses tend to be short courses where the holes are generally 250 feet and shorter. Experienced players tend not to play these courses because they think they are too short or not challenging enough because drivers are not needed. However, these courses are excellent places to practice your midrange throws. As discussed in chapter 3, many of the very best courses feature par-4 and par-5 holes. In essence, each hole on a recreational course can be much like an approach throw on par-4 and par-5 holes. To birdie these longer holes, it is a good idea to practice on short recreational holes. We encourage you to try playing a round by throwing five to seven discs on each hole and tracking the number that land in the circle of love. You could also hole out all five to seven discs and track the number of birdies and pars you carded. Another variation you can try on recreational courses is to play a round by practicing only the throws that need the most improvement.

Great Playing Formats

This section describes in detail two alternatives to the traditional singles, stroke-play format. If you are looking for a standards-based curriculum for the outdoor classroom, we strongly recommend the educational curriculum book *Getting the EDGE*, published by the Educational Disc Golf Experience. It contains a variety of lessons, games, activities, and resource materials designed for students of all ages and abilities.

Doubles Play

If you really want to develop your game, playing in singles, stroke-play tournaments is imperative, but a lot of people choose to play mostly doubles events, and they are also helpful for improving your game. Many people believe that weekly club-sponsored doubles events, or "dubs" as they are often called, are the lifeblood of the sport, and we tend to agree with them. There are many misnomers about what the different doubles games are called. Technically, most disc golf doubles events follow a two-person scramble format, but we are not going to get caught up in what to call it because the word *doubles* refers

to the same basic format at most events. There are special rules for doubles tournaments, but this section summarizes what players should know before showing up to their first weekly doubles event.

Most weekly doubles events feature a cash pot and a random draw. Basically, you throw about five dollars into a hat and then draw a chip or playing card to determine your playing partner. Two-player teams play the course, and the winning pair gets the cash. Sometimes, when a lot of players show up, the payout can be four or more pairs deep, or about one-third of the pool. At larger club events, they may have a stratified random draw in which you may be placed in an *A* pool with advanced players and professionals or a *B* pool with beginners and intermediate players. One playing partner is selected from each pool to form a pair. In this way, two beginners do not end up as partners playing against two experienced players. A lot of players live for the weekly drawing. Will you get a good partner? Will you draw a close friend? Will you have cool people on your card? Just thinking of it can give players goose bumps.

Rules and Strategies

Doubles rules are pretty simple and are nearly identical to the two-person scramble format in traditional golf. On every hole, each playing partner drives from each tee pad. Next, one person in the pair marks where the best throw came to rest with a marker disc. Oftentimes, the best lie is determined by the pair and is typically the one closest to, or with the best line to, the target. Each member of the pair throws his or her next throw from the marker disc, and so on, until one member of the pair holes out. Of course, the scores in doubles events tend to be lower than during singles play, largely because errant shots may not be as penalized. After all, you have a playing partner for a reason—to save you from your dreadful throws.

A lot of people prefer to alternate who drives first on each hole, but this is more a tradition than a rule. Many people prefer to alternate shots as well. For example, if it was your disc that was marked for the next throw, then your partner throws from that spot first. These customs often change if two people of differing skill levels are partners. When in doubt, ask your partner what he or she prefers.

Strategizing during doubles play is really enjoyable, and there are two basic approaches: try to hole out on every throw or lay up for an easy putt. During most rounds, you and your partner will likely try a combination of both strategies, although laying up is far less frequent in doubles play. If you are throwing first, be aggressive but not stupid. If your partner's disc comes to rest out-of-bounds, make every effort to throw your disc in bounds, even if your throw is horribly short. If your partner's throw comes to rest very close to the target, try not to throw short or low. Aim at the top of the target and try to hole out. If your throw had

at least a chance of holing out, you will not likely be criticized. Some people prefer to let the best putter of the pair throw first to increase the odds of either player holing out.

If an odd number of people show up to play dubs, then someone has to play by him- or herself. In Asheville, North Carolina, the local club calls it playing Hans, which is short for Han Solo. Other clubs use different names (in Nashville they call it Clint, for example), but for the solo player, the concept is pretty much the same.

When playing solo, you get one mulligan (or mullie, as it is often called) per hole. A mulligan is a throw that does not count at all, and hence you get to re-throw without penalty. Mulligans do not carry over from one hole to the next, so you cannot save them up if you do not use them. If you re-throw without penalty and your re-throw is worse than your original throw, then you may elect to use your original throw. If your throw comes to rest close enough that you feel you can easily make your putt, then you should use your mulligan. If your disc comes to rest at a place from which you are not very confident you can make your putt, then you have some decision making to do. Saving your mulligans for putts is generally a good idea, but the risk-versus-reward aspect of playing solo is what makes it exciting. Of course, if you are a novice player, you are better off playing with a good partner than playing solo. If you are an experienced player, you might enjoy playing solo because you will have the opportunity to work on your game, you do not have to split the cash prize with a partner, and you can choose to tee off twice on every hole, thus increasing your probability of getting an ace. These basic rules of the game and these simple strategies should get you through your first weekly dubs.

We have three other tips concerning doubles play: One, ask what time the event is likely to finish. If you have another commitment, then do not play. (Nothing is more annoying than having a partner bail in the middle of a round because of another commitment.) Two, bring small bills and a mini marker disc. Three, part with a dollar or two and buy into the ace pool. It is better than going to Vegas. On several occasions we have witnessed the cheerful roar of a group interrupted with the words, "I didn't buy into the ace pool."

Wolf

Wolf can be played with almost any number of players, but it is a great format to play with five people. After all, fivesomes are not frowned upon in disc golf as they are in traditional golf, and it is a great format to play when five friends show up at the local course to play. The rules of Wolf undoubtedly vary, but the version described here is about as universal as it gets. It may seem complicated at first, but it does not take long to figure out once you start playing. The basic rules of disc golf apply, such as holing out, marking your lie, keeping score on each hole, etc. Keep in mind that the example outlined here assumes you are playing with five players.

Winning the Round

Each hole is worth one skin. The hole must be won outright for a skin to be awarded. If the hole is tied, it is called a push, and the next hole is worth two skins and so on. Pushes are common, and thus one hole ultimately can be worth many skins. The pressure of some holes being worth more skins can create some nervous anticipation and entertaining

theater, which makes Wolf, and games like it, really exciting to play.

Number of Holes

As a group, the first decision you have to make is how many holes you want to play. If you are playing with five people, you must play a multiple of five holes (e.g., 10, 15, 20, or 25). We like to play 20 holes on an 18-hole course so the group can play the entire course plus two additional holes. It does not matter on which hole the group begins play, but deciding exactly which holes to play and from which tee pads to play them before you start is a wise practice any time you play disc golf.

Teeing Order

The teeing order in Wolf is pivotal to get correct, but easy to do. First, the group needs to determine the teeing order for the first hole to be played. You can flip discs, draw straws, or determine the order any way the group decides. Once the initial teeing order is set, write it down on a scorecard just as you normally would. For example, let's assume the teeing order is: Eric, Andrew, Clark, Sara, and then Nate. Regardless of the outcome of hole 1, Eric tees off last on hole 2 and the other players move up in the teeing order. So the teeing order for the second hole is Andrew, Clark, Sara, Nate, and then Eric. This is repeated until the end of the round. If done correctly, Eric will tee off first on holes 1, 6, 11, and 16. If you play 20 holes, each person has a chance to tee off first exactly four times during the round, and teeing off first has its advantages in this game.

Strategy

Remember the initial teeing order: Eric, Andrew, Clark, Sara, and then Nate. After Eric drives hole 1 (i.e., after his disc comes to rest) but before Andrew tees off, Eric has a decision to make. If he feels he can win the hole outright playing against the rest of the group, then he howls like a wolf at a full moon: "Oooooowwww!" As you might expect, this spectacle is often rewarded with raucous cheers. The rest of the group then plays a 4-person scramble against Eric. They each get to throw from the best of the four possible lies until someone holes out for the team.

If Eric howls like a wolf and wins the hole (e.g., he cards a birdie and the four-person team cards a par or worse), he earns double the skin value for that hole. In this example, Eric would earn two skins. If Eric loses the hole (e.g., he cards a par and the others card a birdie), then the other four players earn two skins each for that hole. If the hole is tied, it is a push and the next hole will be worth two skins. Rarely, and often in desperation, someone will howl even before they tee off. Called a *blind wolf*, if the player wins the hole outright, he or she earns triple the skin value for that hole. If the blind wolf player loses the hole, the other players earn triple the skin value for that hole. Howling is a big risk that can deliver big rewards. You can only howl on the holes where you tee off first.

After Eric drives on hole 1, if chooses not to howl, he is shopping for a partner. Andrew tees off next, and after his disc comes to rest (but before the next person tees off), Eric must decide if he wants Andrew as his partner for the remainder of hole 1. If Andrew throws a great drive, Eric might choose him. Let's assume Andrew's drive goes horribly awry, and thus Eric decides to wait for a potentially better partner. Clark tees off next, and Eric has the same option: to choose Clark as his partner before the next person tees off, or to wait for a potentially better one. Let's assume he waits. Sara tees off next. If Eric does not announce that he wants Sara as a partner before Nate tees off, then Eric is forced to have Nate as his partner regardless of how Nate throws. Let's assume this happens. For the remainder of hole 1, Eric and Nate will play a two-person scramble against the three-person scramble team of Andrew, Clark, and Sara. The three-person team has the obvious advantage of having three options instead of two from which to throw their next shot. However, since Eric had the opportunity to pick his partner, the odds are good that the pair has at least a decent drive in which to throw from next. If the pair or team of three wins the hole outright, they each get one skin. If the hole is tied, it is a push.

On hole 2, it is Andrew's turn to drive first and he is faced with the same options Eric had on hole 1. It may sound confusing at first, but after you play a couple of holes it becomes easy to follow. Choosing partners, waiting for a potentially better option, playing three players against two, and howling like a lunatic all add to the drama and enjoyment of playing Wolf. Good-natured ribbing or all-out smack talking are often part of the game and are even encouraged. The scoring is not that complicated, but it calls for good record-keeping. Wolf is a great game to play with players of varied skill levels and experience because of its unique problem-solving, risk-taking format.

Manufacturers' Information

We want to acknowledge each of the following manufacturers for helping to grow the sport of disc golf. The manufacturers are presented in alphabetical order, and we only include those manufacturers who agreed to be part of this book. We encourage you to visit their websites to learn more about their companies and their great products.

Disc Golf Association—www.discgolf.com

The Disc Golf Association (DGA) was founded in 1976 by "Steady" Ed Headrick. DGA has a knowledgeable staff of disc golf professionals who and can help guide anyone through the planning, designing, and installation of a disc golf course as well as help with disc selection. Its most popular discs include: Torrent, Hurricane, Squall, Aftershock, Breaker, and Blowfly.

Discraft—www.discraft.com

Discraft was founded in 1978 by Jim Kenner, with an obsessive focus on quality and consistency. Discraft continues to maintain a rock-solid reputation for using engineering-grade polymers and precision craftsmanship. The Discraft

Ultra-Star has been the official disc of USA Ultimate since 1991. Its most popular discs also include: Buzz, Nuke, Soft Banger, Avenger SS, Comet, and Magnet.

Dynamic Discs—www.dynamicdiscs.com

Dynamic Discs got started in the disc golf business in March 2005 and has emerged from a large field of disc golf companies making and selling branded discs and apparel. With the help of talented graphic designers who have produced some distinctive designs, Dynamic Discs has been able to reach out to many disc golfers. The company's most popular discs include: Judge, Truth, Trespass, Escape, Witness, and Verdict.

Gateway Discs—www.gdstour.com

Gateway Discs was founded by David McCormick in 1993, with the intention of growing the sport of disc golf in the St. Louis area. Gateway started manufacturing discs in 1999 and currently has models of golf discs with a wide variety of thermoplastic-engineered polymers. Gateway is well known for its line of putters, which come in a wide range of flexibilities. Its most popular discs include: Wizard, Magic, Assassin, Element, Spirit, and Sabre.

Innova—www.innovadiscs.com

Innova was formed in 1983 by Dave Dunipace, Harold Duvall, and Charlie Duvall. It created the world's first beveled-edge disc designed specifically for disc golf. Innova offers a complete line of precision-molded golf discs to meet the demands of any player's skill level as well as the popular DISCatcher Pro, Sport, and Traveler targets. Its most popular discs include: Aviar, Roc, TeeBird, Valkyrie, Leopard, and Yeti.

Latitude 64°—www.latitude64.se

Latitude 64° is the geographical location of the residential community of Bergsbyn, located outside the coastal city of Skellefteå, near the Arctic Circle in the northeastern part of Sweden. The passionate people behind Latitude 64° are Tomas Ekström, Svante Eriksson, David Berglund, and Johan Åström. Between them, they have been playing disc golf for more than 100 years. Its most popular discs include: Diamond, River, Pure, Saint, Claymore, and Scythe.

Millennium—www.golfdisc.com

Millennium Golf Discs was founded in 1995 by disc golf hall of famers John Houck and Harold Duvall. In 2011, the worldwide distribution and operations of Millennium was taken over by Discs Unlimited in Herington, Kansas. Millennium continues to focus on delivering highly controllable, premium golf discs, as well as growing the sport through course design, awareness, and events. Its most popular discs include: Omega Super Soft, Aurora MS, JLS, Orion LF, Quasar, and Astra.

MVP Disc Sports—www.mvpdiscsports.com

MVP Disc Sports was founded by Chad and Brad Richardson, passionate disc golfers who spent much of their youth working for their father in an injection-molding shop. Avid disc golfers with a drive for perfection, they continue to improve quality, consistency, and performance to the greatest extent possible. Their most popular discs include: Ion, Vector, Volt, Servo, Envy, and Tesla.

Prodigy Disc—www.prodigydisc.com

Prodigy Disc is a unique company founded by a team of world champion disc golfers who felt the need to develop a more consistent golf disc. In its first two years of existence, Prodigy Disc has won more Majors, National Tour tournaments, and PDGA world titles in the open divisions than all the other manufacturers combined. Its most popular discs include: X1, D1, M2, M4, and Pa4.

Vibram—www.vibramdiscgolf.com

Vibram is recognized as the industry leader in the production of high-performance rubber outsoles in the markets of sport, leisure, orthopedic, and work footwear and repair. In 2008, Vibram began applying this knowledge of rubber's capabilities to golf discs. Vibram's X-Link compounds provide excellent grip (especially in bad weather) and incredible durability. Its most popular discs include: VP, Ridge, Ibex, Trak, and Lace.

Glossary

acceleration: The rate of change in velocity.

ace: Achieved when holing out in one throw.

ace pool: Money collected during weekly events or tournaments that goes to the player(s) who score an ace.

advance ratio: Spin rate relative to velocity. Causes a thrown disc to fade.

angle of attack: See *pitch angle*.

anhyzer: A throwing angle in which the outer rim of a disc is tilted upward.

approach throw: A throw in which a player tries to land a disc as close to the target or desired landing area as possible.

away player: The player farthest from the target after all players have driven from the tee pad.

backhand throw: A style of throw in which a player rotates his spine and faces away from the target.

basket: See *target*.

birdie: A score of one throw under par.

blade: A disc thrown at a 90° angle of attack that flies nearly vertical.

blind throw: A throw with no sight line to the target.

bogey: A score of one throw over par.

Bonopane grip: Achieved by placing the rim of the disc in between the index and middle fingers, so the index finger rests on the flight plate and the middle finger is tucked underneath the rim.

casual water: Water that is not considered out-of-bounds, such as puddles or marsh areas.

center of mass: The theoretical point on a flying disc on which gravity acts. Typically the center of a disc.

center of pressure: The theoretical point at which drag and lift forces act on a flying disc.

circle of love: A theoretical circle around a target in which the chances of making a putt are likely.

clown hole: A fluky or puerile hole that often rewards luck over skill.

contextual interference: A learning benefit observed when skills are practiced more at random than repeated.

contralateral stance: Occurs when the lead foot is opposite the throwing hand. Used when throwing forehands and overheads.

crow hop: A type of run-up used when performing overhead throws.

cut roller: A throw that rolls in an upside down *U*-shaped pattern without turning over. Executed by releasing the disc at a hyzer angle.

deuce: A score of 2.

disc: A generic term used to describe the implement used when playing disc golf or Ultimate.

dogleg: A bend in the fairway.

double bird grip: Achieved by placing both the index and pinky fingertips on the inside of the disc rim.

double bogey: A score of two throws over par.

double eagle: A score of three throws under par.

drag: A force that acts in opposition to the relative motion of an object.

drive: A throw executed from a tee pad. The first throw on a given hole.

dual lifetime sport: A sport that requires at least two people to play, such as tennis.

dynamic fluid force: Pressure exerted on a flying disc by air molecules.

eagle: A score of two throws under par.

ego orientation: Perceived ability and success based on the ability and success of other people.

elevator putt: See *loft putt*.

fade: Occurs when a flying disc loses velocity and stability. The tendency of a disc to fly left to right for a right-handed player using a backhand throwing style.

fairway: The indented line of flight or route of a disc on a given hole.

fan grip: Achieved by fanning out the fingers underneath the flat part of the disc, creating more stability in the hand before the release point.

flex shot: A throw that gently turns without losing stability in flight.

flexibility: The capability to move muscles and joints through their full ranges of motion.

flick putt: A forehand-style putt that uses the wrist to create acceleration.

flight plate: The top portion of a disc inside the rim.

flip: See *roll*.

flow: A mental state of operation characterized by feelings of energized focus, full involvement, and enjoyment.

flyway: See *fairway*.

follow-through: All body movement that occurs after a disc is released.

force: Any influence that causes an object to start, stop, speed up, slow down, or change direction.

forehand: A style of throw in which a player rotates the spine but faces the target.

form drag: The sum of the impact forces resulting from the collision between air molecules and a flying disc.

four-finger grip: An alternative to the longhorn grip, used when turbo putting.

fun golf: A casual round in which scores are de-emphasized and enjoyment is the primary objective.

glow golf: A game played at night with glowing discs or lights affixed to discs.

gravity: A constant vertical force defined as the weight of an object.

green: The area around the target from which a putt can be made with few impediments.

grenade: A disc thrown at about a 90° angle that drops almost straight to the ground.

grip: The contact point of a player's hand and a disc.

grip lock: Occurs when a disc is released later than optimal in the throwing motion.

guts: A game in which players throw a disc as fast as possible (so as not to be caught) at an opposing five-person team.

gyroscopic stability: Resistance to angular motion.

hole: Part of a series that constitutes a course. Consists of a tee pad, fairway, green, target, and hazards.

holing out: The act of completing a hole. Achieved when a disc comes to rest in the lower basket assembly or supported by the chains.

hyzer: A throwing angle achieved when outer rim of the disc is tilted downward.

hyzer flip: A disc thrown at a hyzer angle that rolls significantly during flight.

imagery: Occurs when utilizing the senses to create or re-create experiences in the mind.

individual lifetime sport: A sport that can be played by oneself, such as traditional golf.

ipsilateral stance: Occurs when the lead foot is on the same side as the throwing hand. Also known as a homolateral stance.

jail: An area in the rough or trees from which it is very difficult to advance.

jump putt: A throw resembling a putt in which the player leaps toward the target to create momentum.

KanJam: A game that resembles both horseshoes and cornhole, played with a disc.

kinematic chain: A sequence of links constrained by their connection to the other links.

kinetic chain: A chain of events used to produce force.

lie: The spot where a player's disc comes to rest.

lift: A force that acts perpendicular to the relative motion of an object.

loft putt: A putt that flies on an upward trajectory toward the target, then loses elevation as it drops in or near the target. Equivalent to a lob shot in traditional golf.

longhorn grip: A grip used when turbo putting.

mandatory: Constrains the route a thrown or rolled disc may take to the target. A thrown disc must pass to the designated side of the mandatory before the hole is completed.

moment: A measure of a force's tendency to cause an object to rotate about a specific point or axis.

mulligan: A throw that does not count on a person's scorecard.

nicing: Saying "Nice!" or another statement about a player's disc while it is in flight.

object course: A course that utilizes trees, signs, and other objects as targets in lieu of official targets.

out-of-bounds: An area where, if a disc comes to rest, there is a penalty. Bodies of water such as lakes, ponds, and streams are typically out-of-bounds.

overmold: A disc that uses one type of plastic blend for the rim and another for the flight plate.

par: The number of throws an experienced player is expected to need to complete a hole.

PDGA Player Rating: A number that indicates how close a player's average round scores are compared to the course rating. A rating of 1,000 is considered a professional-caliber round.

penalty throw: A throw assessed when a disc comes to rest out-of-bounds, a mandatory is missed, or another rule violation has occurred.

perceived competence: A person's expectation of achieving success.

percentage of open space: The percent of airspace available for a potential flight path or route.

pitch angle: A disc's back-to-front tilt relative to its direction of flight.

pitch putt: A putting style that uses leg flexion and extension to propel the disc with little spin.

Pluto Platter: The first Walter Fredrick Morrison–designed disc sold by Wham-O Mfg. Co.

Pole-hole: "Steady" Ed Headrick's landmark three-dimensional target.

power grip: Achieved by placing four fingers on the inside lip of the disc. Used to create leverage and power while driving.

provisional throw: An additional throw not added to a player's score if it is not ultimately used in completion of the hole. Most often used when there is a better-than-average chance a player's disc is lost or out-of-bounds.

pull-through: The phase of throwing from the end of the reach back to the release point.

push putt: A putting style that uses leg extension and shoulder abduction to propel the disc on a low-to-high flight line.

putt: A throwing style used when a player is close enough to the target to hole out.

quarterwind: A combination of a headwind or tailwind and a crosswind.

reach-back: The phase of throwing executed by extending the throwing arm away from the intended line of flight.

ready golf: A style of play in which the away player rule is disregarded, particularly used when putting.

Ring of Fire: An elimination game in which many players putt at the same time at the same target.

roll: A moment that acts on a flying disc. Also called *flip* or *turn*.

roller: A throw designed to fly for a short distance and then land on the ground and roll like a wheel.

rotary force: See *torque.*

route: Gaps between trees and other hazards that delineate where a player's thrown disc should navigate to reach the green or landing area in the fairway.

safari golf: A game in which players choose holes other than an established layout.

Saucer Golf: Indicates disc golf played on courses that use rare cone-shaped targets.

Scratch Scoring Average: A metric of course difficulty based on what scratch players scored during a given round. Players rated 1,000 are considered scratch players.

seasoned disc: A disc that has been worn by being thrown repeatedly or by sanding.

sidearm: See *forehand.*

skins: A game in which each hole is played separately. A skin is earned by the player with the lowest score on the hole. In the event of a tie, the skin carries over to the next hole.

sky roller: A throw that flies in the air for a significant distance before it turns over, hits the ground on a vertical angle, and begins to roll.

speed: A rating of a disc's overall drag coefficient.

speed golf: A game in which the object is to play a round as fast as possible or with some combination of time and score.

spike hyzer: A disc thrown at a severe hyzer angle and high in the air.

spin: Rotation around an axis.

spin putt: A style of putt in which the goal is to spin the disc.

split finger grip: Commonly used when executing a forehand throwing style.

S-shot: A snake-like disc flight that initially turns, then fades.

stance: The contact point of a player and the ground. Typically established with the feet.

straddle stance: A putting stance in which the player's feet are about parallel with his or her shoulders.

stroke average: The mean score on a given hole. Used to estimate the difficulty of a given hole.

surface drag: The sum of the friction forces acting between the air molecules and the surface of a disc or the friction forces between the air molecules themselves.

target: The equivalent of the hole/pin/flag combination in traditional golf.

target golf: A game in which trees, signs, and other objects are used instead of a standard target.

task orientation: Occurs when perceptions of ability and success are self-referenced.

tee pad: A designed area from which players must drive the disc. Typically constructed of concrete or grass.

throwing angle: A disc's side-to-side tilt immediately before release.

thumber: A style of throw similar to throwing a baseball or softball. Tumbles from right to left when thrown by a right-handed player.

tomahawk: A style of throw similar to throwing a baseball or softball. Tumbles from left to right when thrown by a right-handed player.

tombstone: A disc partially buried in the ground.

torque: The turning effect produced by a force.

tournament director: The person in charge of enforcing the rules of play during a tournament.

turbo putt: A style of putt achieved by releasing the disc at or above the shoulders using your wrist and forearm to spin the disc.

turbulent flow: A highly irregular configuration of air molecules that creates drag.

turn: The tendency of a flying disc to gently roll about its axis. The equivalent to a draw in traditional golf.

two-step approach: Used to create momentum and rhythm when executing approach throws.

Ultimate: A team field game that resembles soccer played with a disc.

unified finger grip: A common forehand grip used to created leverage.

upshot: See *approach throw*.

vector: A mathematical representation of anything described by both its magnitude and direction.

velocity: The magnitude and direction of motion represented by a vector.

Wolf: A playing format typically played with four or five people.

X-step: A series of steps used to create momentum and align the hips perpendicular to the intended target.

Notes

Chapter 2

future sales of flying discs Feidt, Joe. Interview by Justin Menickelli, March 23, 2014.

Frisbee should not be overlooked Palmeri, Jim and Joe Feidt. "How a Humble Newsletter Connected the Frisbee World." *Disc Golfer* (Winter 2012): 36–38.

make their citywide event a national tournament Palmieri, Jim. Interview by Justin Menickelli, October 16, 2011.

because it was simply a better target Feidt, Joe. "The Birth of Innova: How Dave Dunipace Dreamed Up and Built a Better Golf Disc." *Disc Golfer* (Summer 2010): 30–31.

Puppy was considered by many to be Feidt, Joe. "The Puppy Master: How Jan 'Whizbo' Sobel Changed Disc Golf Forever." *Disc Golfer* (Winter 2011): 44–47.

first coined by Roddick Palmieri & Feidt, "How a Humble Newsletter Connected the Frisbee World," 36–38.

locally brewed Genesee Cream Ale Feidt, Joe. "It was 30 Years Ago Today: How One Seismic Year Shook Disc Golf." *Disc Golfer* (Summer 2013): 48–51.

more than $2 million has been raised Interview by Justin Menickelli.

less than 10 percent of disc golf courses are private Oldakowski, Rau and John W. McEwen. "Diffusion of Disc Golf Courses in the United States." *Geographical Review* (July 2013): 355–71.

can easily exceed $500,000 Moore, James Francis. "Building and Maintaining the Truly Affordable Golf Course." USGA. http://www.usga.org /course_care/articles/construction/general /Building-And-Maintaining-The-Truly -Affordable-Golf-Course. Accessed May 2015.

Chapter 3

Houck calls a dumb hole Houck, John. Interview by Justin Menickelli. September 21, 2011.

it can be called dumb luck Ibid.

more closely resemble great traditional golf courses Ibid.

"I can't throw from here?" Houck, John. "Making Something from Nothing Is a Tall Order." *Disc Golfer* (Winter 2015): 61–64.

where the fairway ends Houck, John. "Building a Better Miss Trap." *Disc Golfer* (Winter 2013): 50–52.

key to the mental part of the game Ibid.

most skillful performance earn the best scores Houck, John. Interview by Justin Menickelli.

Chapter 5

Gallwey explains the performance triangle Gallwey, Timothy. *The Inner Game of Golf.* New York: Random House, 1998.

effort, persistence, satisfaction, and performance Duda, J.L. "Sport and exercise motivation: A goal perspective analysis." In *Motivation in Sport and Exercise.* Ed. G. Roberts. Champaign, IL: Human Kinetics. 1992: 57–91.

can undoubtedly and consistently increase performance Gould, Dan. "Goal Setting for Peak Performance." In *Applied Sport Psychology: Personal Growth to Peak Performance*, edited by Jean Williams, 190–205. Mountain View, CA: Mayfield Publishing, 2001.

Chapter 7

drag and lift can be considered conventionally Lorenz, Ralph. "Flying Saucers." *New Scientist* (June 2004): 40–41.

overall thickness can also have profound effects Kamaruddin, Noorfazreena. "Dynamics and Performance of Flying Discs." Dissertation, University of Manchester, 2011. https://www.escholar.manchester.ac.uk/uk-ac-man-scw:132975

connected to the surface as long as possible Hummel, Sarah. "Frisbee Flight Simulation and Throw Biomechanics." MSC thesis, UC Davis, 2003. http://biosport.ucdavis.edu/research-projects/frisbee-flight-simulation-and-throw-biomechanics/HummelThesis.pdf

pitching is significantly reduced during flight Lorenz, Ralph. "Flying Saucers," 40–41.

significant effect on lift-to-drag ratio Kamaruddin, Noorfazreena. "Dynamics and Performance of Flying Discs."

exhibit minimal roll about the flight axis Ibid.

the COP moves accordingly Hummel, "Frisbee Flight Simulation and Throw Biomechanics" and Hummel, Sarah and Mont Hubbard. "Implications of Frisbee Dynamics and Aerodynamics on Possible Flight Patterns." In *The Engineering of Sport* 5, edited by M. Hubbard, R.D.

divergence from optimal release conditions Kamaruddin, Noorfazreena. "Dynamics and Performance of Flying Discs."

drivers can fly about 12 percent Ibid.

Chapter 13

take advantage of a contextual interference effect Shea, J.B. and R.L. Morgan. "Contextual Interference Effects on the Acquisition, Retention and Transfer of a Motor Skill." *Journal of Experimental Psychology: Human Learning and Memory* 5 (1979): 179–87

Sources

Bloomfield, Louis. "Working Knowledge on the Flight of the Frisbee." *Scientific American* (April 1999).

Caney, Steven. "The Invention of the Frisbee." In *Steven Caney's Invention Book*, 97–102. New York: Workman Publishing Co., Inc., 1999.

Convers, Ron and Brendan Hicks. "Mastering the Wind." Discraft. Accessed October 2013. http://www.discraft.com/res_wind06_p1.html.

Duda, J.L. "Sport and Exercise Motivation: A Goal Perspective Analysis." In *Motivation in Sport and Exercise*. Ed. G. Roberts. Champaign, IL: Human Kinetics. 1992: 57–91.

Duvall, Harold. Interview by Justin Menickelli. September 19, 2011.

Feidt, Joe. "The Birth of Innova: How Dave Dunipace Dreamed Up and Built a Better Golf Disc." *Disc Golfer* (Summer 2010): 30–31.

———. "Creativity Unchained: How Ed and Ken Headrick Invented the Disc Golf Pole Hole." *Disc Golfer* (Summer 2012): 26–29.

———. Interview by Justin Menickelli. March 23, 2014.

———. "It was 30 Years Ago Today: How One Seismic Year Shook Disc Golf." *Disc Golfer* (Summer 2013): 48–51.

———. "Kaboom: Five Big Bangs That Launched Disc Golf." *Disc Golfer* (Summer 2012): 14–16.

———. "The Puppy Master: How Jan 'Whizbo' Sobel Changed Disc Golf Forever." *Disc Golfer* (Winter 2011): 44–47.

———. "25 Years of Ice Bowl." *Disc Golfer* (Spring 2011): 22–26.

Finley, Holly. Interview by Justin Menickelli. March 5, 2014.

Gallwey, Timothy. *The Inner Game of Golf.* New York: Random House, 1998.

Gould, Dan. "Goal Setting for Peak Performance." In *Applied Sport Psychology: Personal Growth to Peak Performance*, edited by Jean Williams, 190–205. Mountain View, CA: Mayfield Publishing, 2001.

Govang, Patrick. Interview by Justin Menickelli. March 11, 2014.

Graham, Brian. Interview by Justin Menickelli. November 1, 2011

Gregory, Michael Stevens. *Disc Golf.* Duluth, MN: Trellis Publishing, Inc., 2003.

Gregory, Sean. "Spin Doctors: Ultimate Frisbee Chucks Its Hippie Past to Go Pro." *Time* (October 7, 2013): 59–66.

Headrick, Edward. Flying Saucer Patent Application No. 3359678. Patented December 26, 1967.

Houck, John. "Building a Better Miss Trap." *Disc Golfer* (Winter 2013): 50–52.

———. "Dumb Holes." HouckDesign. Accessed September 2012. http://www.houckdesign.com/dumbholes.html

———. Interview by Justin Menickelli. September 21, 2011.

———. "The Long and Winding Route." *Disc Golfer* (Fall 2013): 56–58.

———. "Making Something from Nothing Is a Tall Order." *Disc Golfer* (Winter 2015): 61–64.

Hummel, Sarah. "Frisbee Flight Simulation and Throw Biomechanics." MSC thesis, UC Davis, 2003. http://biosport.ucdavis.edu/research-projects/frisbee-flight-simulation-and-throw-biomechanics/HummelThesis.pdf

Hummel, Sarah and Mont Hubbard. "Implications of Frisbee Dynamics and Aerodynamics on Possible Flight Patterns." In *The Engineering of Sport* 5, edited by M. Hubbard, R.D. Mehta, and J.M. Pallis, 407–13. M. Hubbard, R.D. Mehta & J.M. Pallis (Eds.), Vol. 1, 407–13, Central Plain Book Mfg., 2004.

Jenkins, Valerie. Interview by Justin Menickelli. August 19, 2013.

Johnson, Stancil. *Frisbee: A Practitioner's Manual and Definitive Treatise*. New York: Workman Publishing Company, 1975.

Kamaruddin, Noorfazreena. "Dynamics and Performance of Flying Discs." Dissertation University of Manchester, 2011. https://www.escholar.manchester.ac.uk/uk-ac-man-scw:132975

Kapalko, Rick. "The 19th Hole." Disc Golfer (Summer 2011), 64.

Kasper, Bob, "Ultimate Frisbee Freaks," *Washington Post*, August 11, 1977, D9–10.

Keasey, Scott. Interview by Justin Menickelli. May 7, 2015.

King, Elaine. Interview by Justin Menickelli. April 24, 2014.

Koon, Bruce, "How to Keep Sales of a Toy Up: Build a Sport Around It," *Wall Street Journal*, August 17, 1979, 19.

Leonardo, Anthony. *Ultimate: The Greatest Sport Ever Invented by Man*. New York: Breakaway Books, 2007.

Loomis, D. "Juliana Kourver Tells How She Discovered Disc Golf, What It Takes to Win, and Why She Walked Away from the Sport." *Disc Golfer* (Winter 2013): 34–38.

Lorenz, Ralph. "Flying Saucers." *New Scientist* (June 2004): 40–41.

———. *Spinning Flight Dynamics of Frisbees, Boomerangs, Samaras, and Skipping Stones*. New York: Springer Science+Business Media, 2010.

Lyksett, Jon. Interview by Justin Menickelli. March 12, 2014.

Malafronte, Victor A. *The Complete Book of Frisbee: The History of the Sport & the First Official Price Guide*. Oceanside, CA: American Trends Publishing Co., 1998.

Martin, Douglas. "Ed Headrick, Designer of the Modern Frisbee, Dies at 78." *New York Times*, August 14, 2002.

McCormack, Dave. Interview by Justin Menickelli. March 7, 2014.

Menickelli, Justin. "Disc Golf Walking Benefits." PDGA. Accessed November 2012. http://www .pdga.com/disc-golf-walking-benefits.html.

———. "A Good Walk Defined: Research Study on Disc Golf Yields Interesting Findings." PDGA. Accessed November 2010. http://www .pdga.com/a-good-walk-defined.html.

Moore, James Francis. "Building and Maintaining the Truly Affordable Golf Course." USGA. http://www.usga.org/course_care/articles /construction/general/Building-And -Maintaining-The-Truly-Affordable-Golf -Course. Accessed May 2015.

Morrison, Fred and Phil Kennedy. *Flat Flip Flies Straight!: True Origins of the Frisbee.* Wethersfield, CT: Wormhole Press, 2006.

Morrison, V.R. "The Physics of Frisbees." *Electronic Journal of Classical Mechanics and Relativity* (April 2005): 1–11.

Norton, Goldy. *The Official Frisbee Handbook.* New York: Bantam Books, 1972.

Oldakowski, Rau and John W. McEwen. "Diffusion of Disc Golf Courses in the United States." *Geographical Review* (July 2013): 355–71.

Palmeri, Jim. "Collecting the Pluto Platter." *Flying Disc* (February 1980): 18–22.

———. Interview by Justin Menickelli. October 16, 2011.

———. "The Space Saucer." *Flying Disc* (April/ May 1980): 46–47.

Palmeri, Jim and Joe Feidt. "How a Humble Newsletter Connected the Frisbee World." *Disc Golfer* (Winter 2012): 36–38.

Pierson, Snapper. Interview by Justin Menickelli. September 23, 2011.

Potts, Jonathan and William Crowther. "Frisbee Aerodynamics." Paper presented at the 20th AIAA Applied Aerodynamics Conference and Exhibit, St. Louis, Missouri (June 2002): 1–14.

The Professional Disc Golf Association. "PDGA Approved Discs." Accessed September 2013. http://www.pdga.com/tech-standards.

———. "Current Disciplinary Actions." Accessed September 2013. http://www.pdga.com /documents/disciplinary-actions.

———. "Official Rules of Disc Golf." Accessed September 2013. http://www.pdga.com/rules /official-rules-disc-golf.

Reading, Des. Interview by Justin Menickelli. February 11, 2014.

Reading, Jay. Interview by Justin Menickelli. June 18, 2013.

Roddick, Dan. *Frisbee Disc Basics.* New York: Prentice Hall, Inc., 1980.

———. Interview by Justin Menickelli. February 18, 2014.

Rothstein, Rick. "Ice Bowl Closes in on 25 Years and Is Bigger than Ever." *Disc Golfer.* Fall 2010: 44-45.

———. Interview by Justin Menickelli. September 26, 2011.

Sappenfield, George. Interview by Justin Menickelli. March 4, 2014.

Shea, J.B. and R.L. Morgan. "Contextual Interference Effects on the Acquisition, Retention and Transfer of a Motor Skill." *Journal of Experimental Psychology: Human Learning and Memory* 5 (1979): 179–87

Sullivan, Brian. Interview by Justin Menickelli. March 3, 2014.

Tips, Charles and Dan Roddick. *Frisbee Sports and Games.* Berkeley, CA: Celestial Arts, 1979.

Tuten, Chris and Justin Menickelli. "Eight Keys to Teaching Disc Golf." *Disc Golfer*. Summer 2012: 56–57.

Vealey, Robin S. and Christy A. Greenleaf. "Seeing is Believing: Understanding and Using Imagery in Sport." In *Applied Sport Psychology: Personal Growth to Peak Performance*, edited by Jean Williams, 247–72. Mountain View, CA: Mayfield Publishing, 2001.

About the Authors

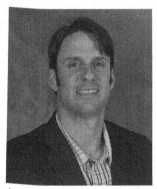

Justin Menickelli. *Photo courtesy of Western Carolina University*

Justin Menickelli is an associate professor at Western Carolina University, where he teaches courses in motor behavior, sports psychology, research methods, and beginning disc golf. He earned a PhD in Kinesiology from Louisiana State University, an MAED in Physical Education from Western Carolina University, and a BS in Exercise Science from SUNY Cortland. He has published numerous articles about disc golf, received several grants to fund disc golf workshops, and designed courses for college campuses and public schools. In 2015 Justin was presented the Educational Disc Golf Experience Award by the PDGA in recognition for teaching disc golf to young people and growing the sport. When not playing, teaching, or writing about disc golf, he enjoys mountain biking and alpine skiing. Justin lives in Cullowhee, North Carolina, with his wife, Kristin; two sons, Aidan and Noah; and daughter, Addison.

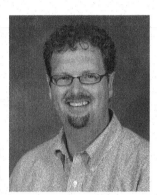

Ryan Pickens. *Photo courtesy of Western Carolina University*

Ryan Pickens earned an MA in Organizational Development and Transformation from the California Institute of Integral Studies and a BS in Human and Organizational Development from Vanderbilt University. In 2012 he finished in the top 25 in the Pro Master's Division at the Disc Golf World Championships. He taught disc golf for a decade at Mars Hill University, has designed two courses in western North Carolina, and is designing several other courses (www.discgolfdesigngroup.com). Currently, he is a full-time strategy and organizational development specialist with Center for Meaningful Work, LLC (www.workwithmeaning.com). When not playing or designing courses, he enjoys freshwater and saltwater fishing. Ryan lives in Asheville, North Carolina, with his wife, Kelly, and daughter, Ellora Don.